The
Medicare
Billing
Troubleshooter
for Clinical Trials

Bill Sarraille, JD
Allison Weber Shuren, MSN, JD

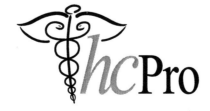

The Medicare Billing Troubleshooter for Clinical Trials is published by HCPro, Inc.

Copyright 2004 HCPro, Inc.

ISBN: 1-57839-317-5

HCPro provides information resources for the health care industry. A selected listing of other newsletters books and other HCPro products is found in the back of this book.

HCPro is not affiliated in any way with the Joint Commission on Accreditation of Healthcare Organizations, which owns the JCAHO trademark.

Bill Sarraille, JD and Allison Weber Shuren, MSN, JD, Authors
Kelly Bilodeau, Managing Editor
Jean St. Pierre, Creative Director
Mike Mirabello, Senior Graphic Artist
Matthew Sharpe, Cover Designer
Leah Tracosas, Senior Copy Editor
John Leonard, Senior Managing Editor
Paul Nash, Group Publisher
Suzanne Perney, Publisher
Holley Thames Lutz, partner, Gardner Carton and Douglas, reviewer

Contributions to the book were also made by Christine A. Jochim, legal assistant
Sidley Austin Brown & Wood LLP

Note: The review provided by Ms. Lutz is not intended as legal advice.

Advice given is general. Readers should consult professional counsel for specific legal, ethical, or clinical questions.

Arrangements can be made for quantity discounts.

For more information, contact:

HCPro
P.O. Box 1168
Marblehead, MA 01945
Telephone: 800/650-6787 or 781/639-1872
Fax: 781/639-2982
E-mail: *customerservice@hcpro.com*

Visit HCPro at its World Wide Web sites:
www.hcmarketplace.com, www.hcpro.com, and *www.himinfo.com*

Contents

Contents

About the Authors

Bill Sarraille, JD

Bill Sarraille, JD, is a partner at the national law firm Sidley Austin Brown & Wood LLP. He is a member of the firm's Health Care Practice Group and concentrates on health care matters, including clinical research trial–related issues. Sarraille has counseled clients on billing, coverage, fraud and abuse, financial relationship, conflicts of interest, internal investigation, False Claims Act, kickback, appropriations and federal grant, IRB, informed consent, HIPAA privacy and security, and many other issues related to research. His clients include hospitals, pharmaceutical companies, health systems, device and equipment manufacturers, faculty practice plans, ambulatory surgical centers, physician practice management companies, managed care organizations, and a number of health care trade associations and professional societies. Sarraille graduated cum laude from Yale University in 1985 and received his law degree from Harvard University in 1989. He is the author of more than three dozen books and articles on billing, coverage, and clinical research issues.

Allison Weber Shuren, MSN, JD

Allison Weber Shuren, MSN, JD, is a senior associate in the Health Law Group at Arent Fox Kintner Plotkin & Kahn, P.L.L.C. Shuren focuses her practice on regulatory and legislative health care matters including

Medicare coverage, reimbursement, and overpayment matters; all aspects of industry-sponsored and federally-funded human subject research compliance; development of clinical research consortiums, fraud, abuse, and False Claims Act counseling and defense for all types of health care providers and pharmaceutical and medical device manufacturers; the HIPAA privacy standards; and issues related to telemedicine and e-health. She advises a diverse group of clients, including hospitals and academic medical centers, physician practices, ambulatory surgery centers, diagnostic imaging centers, health care professional societies, pharmaceutical and medical device companies, and internet-based health care companies. Shuren has testified before the U.S. House Energy and Commerce Subcommittee on Health regarding Medicare Part B fee schedule payment policy.

Shuren also is a critical care clinical nurse specialist and pediatric nurse practitioner with a specialty in pediatric cardiology, cardiovascular surgery and neonatal surgery. She has served as a clinical trials coordinator as well as a principal investigator. Shuren received her law degree from the University of Michigan, an MS in nursing from the University of Florida, and a bachelor's degree in nursing from Salem (MA) State College.

Guide to acronyms

You will notice that this book uses several common acronyms. Although each one is spelled out the first time it is used, you may find this list a help-ful reference as you read.

AHRQ: Agency for Healthcare Research and Quality

CDC: Centers for Disease Control and Prevention

CMS: Centers for Medicare and Medicaid Services (formerly known as HCFA)

DOD: Department of Defense

DOJ: Department of Justice

FDA: U.S. Food and Drug Administration

FI: fiscal intermediary

HIPAA: Health Insurance Portability and Accountability Act of 1996

IDE: investigational device exemption

IND: investigational new drug

LMRP: local medical review policy

NCD: national coverage decision

NIH: National Institutes of Health

VA: Department of Veterans Affairs

Introduction

The Medicare Billing Troubleshooter for Clinical Trials is designed to help your research organization understand the complex regulations related to Medicare billing for clinical trials. It was written for those on the front lines of billing—the billing and finance professionals, compliance officers, investigators, and research coordinators—who need to know how to get accurate payments for services related to clinical trials. It's not an easy job.

Medicare's clinical research billing laws have recently undergone significant changes: Within the past three years, the Medicare program has shifted from providing limited support for research to offering significant reimbursement for clinical trial–related services.

These rapid changes have led to ambiguity and confusion. Even organizations that understand the regulations may have difficulty applying them in practical terms. And misunderstandings can be costly. The government has been cracking down hard on violations related to clinical trials, in some cases doling out multimillion-dollar fines to institutions that it contends have violated Medicare fraud and abuse laws.

This book can help you avoid placing your facility at risk. It will focus on practical, procedural issues to help you apply the billing regulations to real-life situations, and it will offer solutions to compliance and implementation

Introduction

challenges. This book will also give you a history of cases and investigations related to improper billing so you can learn from the mistakes of your colleagues. The challenges they faced are ones you are bound to encounter.

CHAPTER 1

An Historic Look at Medicare Billing for Clinical Trials

Chapter 1

An Historic Look at Medicare Billing for Clinical Trials

In the past, if you were looking to bill Medicare for items or services related to clinical trials, you were pretty much out of luck. The only time Medicare would pay for clinical trial–related costs was if the subject of a clinical trial had experienced complications during participation, and if it was the type of ailment that Medicare would ordinarily cover. In other words, Medicare allowed providers to bill for items or services used as part of diagnosis or treatment of complications.

Let's consider an example: A patient was admitted to a hospital for an experimental transplant service. Historically, Medicare would pay neither for the transplant surgery itself nor the related hospital care. The organization that sponsored the clinical trial research would have to pay for these services and items, or payment would have to come from the patient, or from the patient's other insurance sources (in the unlikely event that the other insurers covered these services or items). As a last option—and the least attractive from the perspective of the providers, of course—the providers would pay for the services themselves by "eating" the costs involved.

Now let's assume that post-discharge, the human subject's immune system rejects the transplanted organ, and complications result. Even under its historic "hands-off" policy with respect to clinical research trials issues, the Medicare program would pay for the services and items that were reasonable and necessary to address the patient's complications.

Further, let's say that our unfortunate transplant patient broke his or her leg walking around the hospital during the recuperation period before discharge. Medicare would pay for those reasonable and necessary services to treat the patient's broken leg. Medicare would pay because it would consider the broken leg "unrelated" to the noncovered clinical research trial services and items.

All in all, Medicare's past support for clinical research was negligible at best. With both experimental items /services and any "related" items/services considered noncovered, the vast majority of costs for clinical trials research fell squarely on sponsoring organizations, research sites, the subjects of the research, and those few third-party payers that adopted a substantially different policy from the Medicare program.

Calls for change

A broad coalition of interest groups—pharmaceutical companies, device manufacturers, academic medical centers, research facilities, and patient advocacy groups—began to lobby for greater Medicare coverage of clinical research trials. They argued that increased federal support for clinical research was necessary to meet increasing demand, to speed the delivery of new technology into the health care system, and to increase the ability of researchers to study "neglected" diseases and conditions—areas where industry sponsorship was likely to be limited.

Two significant developments followed. The first was the creation of coverage for certain device-oriented research. On November 1, 1995, the government established a process that allowed Medicare to cover services related to some medical devices that were formerly refused coverage as experimental.

In order to qualify for coverage, a device must be

- in Category B, under FDA regulations, which means it is safe, effective, and nonexperimental

- used in an Food and Drug Administration (FDA)–approved trial

- medically necessary

We discuss this coverage in greater detail in the chapters that follow. Though advocates of government support of clinical trials research hailed the introduction of this coverage, the change was greeted with grumbling that it only represented a first step toward the support that was needed.

Pharmaceutical manufacturers, in particular, said they had been "left out in the cold" because device manufacturers were the only entities eligible for the expanded coverage.

The second major development occurred on June 7, 2000, when President Clinton issued an executive order that authorized the Centers for Medicare & Medicaid Services (CMS) to pay "routine costs" for patients in qualified clinical trials. A national coverage decision (NCD) followed that memorandum and, as of September 19, 2000, some items or services "related" to clinical trials became eligible for coverage under Medicare.

The 2000 NCD marked a strategic and quite political compromise. The Clinton administration, by authorizing some reimbursement for clinical trials, seized the opportunity to curry favor with industry and special interest groups, as well as patients. Yet it did so with a coverage rule that did not offer expanded coverage for experimental items or services. And coverage for routine care was only offered to a limited number of facilities. As a result, some advocates of clinical research expressed their disappointment that the Clinton administration's policy did not go far enough; however, most enthusiastically welcomed the change.

Coverage stirs controversy

Some within CMS did not support the new policy. They claimed that the expansion of coverage constituted bad policy because it placed additional burdens on a fiscally shaky Medicare program. The dissenters at CMS and in Congress argued that the costs of clinical research should be borne by the private marketplace. According to these critics of the policy, shareholders of pharmaceutical, device, and equipment manufacturers, biotech companies, and venture capital funds should pay for the costs of clinical research, as they do with other research and development costs.

At least some of the well-publicized reluctance among critics at CMS to embrace the Clinton administration's policy can be traced. For example, some dissenters claimed the administration was heavy-handed and that the supporters allegedly "forced" the policy onto the agency, an action that ruffled feathers (and egos). Some critics at CMS felt that the coverage issue was symbolic of the agency's perceived woes, perceiving CMS as caught between an overly intrusive administration and a micromanaging Congress.

To some extent, concerns about the prospect of administering the coverage policy also underlay the CMS opposition. The dissenters wanted to help improve care for those whose only hope for a cure might come through research, but they feared that implementing the NCD would be a nightmare from an administrative standpoint, particularly if the full range of trials that the NCD could support was made eligible for coverage. Concerns about overtaxing CMS' budget and human resources crept into the debate.

Taking a step back, the extension of coverage to clinical trials raised the basic question, what should the Medicare program pay for? Should Medicare help develop new technology? Or should the program simply try to provide a reasonable level of care for patients using whatever technology the health care industry has been able to bring to market with the level of support that the federal government has traditionally given through the National Institutes of Health (NIH) and other granting agencies? The debate on this point continues today, as advocates for clinical research support continue to push for expanded coverage.

The present and future of coverage

Medicare's expansion of coverage to date has measurably improved the amount of clinical research that can be conducted. The number of trials has exploded in recent years. That explosion in clinical research is, at least in part, a function of expanded Medicare coverage and the program's support of clinical trials via reimbursement. In fact, at this point, an increasingly significant issue in clinical research is the shortage of human participants.

However, even with its successes the current coverage environment is far from ideal—both advocates and opponents of expanded coverage agree on that. The regulations regarding clinical trials coverage may have changed, but the patchwork of coverage, the ambiguity and pitfalls present in the coverage rules, and the corresponding billing and coding requirements have given critics much fodder.

It may surprise some, but many critics remain opposed to the decision to extend coverage to clinical trials. Clinical trials coverage is closely tied to anti-pharmaceutical company rhetoric that accompanies such hotly debated proposals as changing payments based on an average wholesale price, developing a Medicare pharmaceutical benefit, and reconsidering the ban on re-importation of pharmaceuticals. Critics argue that Medicare support of trials is supposedly permitting pharmaceutical companies to avoid costs they should bear, given the profits that they receive once a successful product hits the market.

Only time will tell how the reimbursement policy will evolve and whether the NCD will be fully implemented. However, it is unlikely that any existing coverage will be curtailed in the absence of some immediate threat to Medicare's viability.

Indeed, as we write this, Congress is debating a Medicare reform bill that would expand clinical research support further. In 2000, CMS said it would implement a presidential executive order to provide reimbursement for the routine costs of care for breakthrough medical technologies, but it has yet to finalize this policy.

Many of the overlooked trials are addressed in a bill introduced in 2003 by representatives Jim Ramstad (R-MN), Anna Eshoo (D-CA), and Joseph Pitts (R-PA) called the Medicare Innovation and Responsiveness Act of 2003. If the bill passes, it would expand coverage of routine costs of clinical trials for investigational devices. It will be interesting—and telling—to see where this proposal ends up.

CHAPTER 2

Device Trials—Two Options for Payment

Chapter 2

Device Trials—Two Options for Payment

Obtaining Medicare coverage for items and services related to device trials is more tedious than getting coverage for pharmaceuticals because Medicare determines device coverage and payment on a case-by-case basis. However, device trials do reap some benefits. For example, device trial coverage includes payment for the investigational device itself. Also, depending on the source of funding for the device trial, it may be eligible for coverage under the device-specific rules or the NCD, while pharmaceutical trials only are eligible for coverage under the NCD. Organizations may opt to pursue coverage under one or the other methodology for eligible device trials, but may not submit claims under both simultaneously.

In 1995, Congress passed a law that allowed services related to the use of certain medical device trials to be covered by Medicare. Before this law, Medicare denied payment for medical devices that had yet to be cleared for marketing by the FDA. The program also denied payment for the services related to their use, under the guise that they were experimental. Congress wanted to make new devices available to beneficiaries, but it did not want Medicare to pay for devices that had not yet been shown to be safe and effective. So Congress required Medicare and the FDA to identify those devices that, although still under clinical trial, were very similar to existing technology known to be safe and effective.

The system decided upon by Medicare requires the FDA to categorize every new device it reviews as either a Category A device or a Category B device. Medicare only pays for services related to certain clinical trials involving Category B devices. Category B devices have an investigational device exemption, or "IDE," from the FDA. Under an IDE, the device goes through a streamlined FDA review. The device is considered so similar to other devices on the market that regulators believe it is at least as safe and effective as these devices, even though they are still subject to human subject clinical trials. On the other hand, Category A devices do not have a functional equivalent that has already been proven to be safe and effective, and, therefore, are considered experimental.

Local Medicare contractors, known as carriers and fiscal intermediaries (FIs), are responsible for determining, case-be-case, whether Medicare will pay for services related to a device clinical trial. To help the contractors decide, Medicare has outlined a number of criteria that must be met in order for them to approve payment. These criteria include the following:

- Use of the device must be part of an FDA-approved clinical trial

- The device must be assigned to Category B as described by FDA regulations

- Use of the device must be medically necessary for the patient for whom coverage is sought

- The amount, duration, and frequency of the use of the device must be medically appropriate

- The device must be used in a setting appropriate for the patient's medical needs and condition

When contractors decide whether to pay for services related to Category B devices, Medicare also directs them to consider any national or local medical coverage policies regarding similar FDA-approved devices. Contractors must also consider any policy, position statements, or recommendations from pertinent national or local health care societies, as well as published reports in respected peer-reviewed journals.

Providers seeking reimbursement bear the burden of ensuring that the contractor has all the necessary information to determine coverage and payment. Thus, if you know you will be seeking payment for services in relation to a device clinical trial, be proactive: Assemble all the necessary background and supportive materials to be submitted to your carrier or FI well before enrolling your first patient in a trial.

Coverage and payment

What will Medicare pay for?

Under the device-trial coverage policy, the device itself and the routine costs associated with its use are eligible for payment. Reimbursement for the device, however, may not exceed the amount Medicare would pay for a comparable device that has already been approved or cleared for marketing by the FDA. Medicare will also pay for the associated routine costs of trial preparation, service furnished along with and necessary to the use of the device, and aftercare services for recovery from the use of the device or from receiving related services. In addition, Medicare will pay for services it would ordinarily reimburse to treat a condition or complication that arises from the use of the Category B device or a related service.

What won't Medicare pay for?

To avoid submitting improper claims to the government, understand what services related to a Category B device trial Medicare will not pay for. Improper claims could lead to a Medicare audit and could lead to allegations that you have submitted false claims to the government. The individuals with responsibility for claims submission must have clear guidelines as to what services may be billed to the program and what may not. We refer to these as billing guidelines. The clinical trial investigator, an experienced member of your billing staff, and your compliance officer should develop these guidelines. New guidelines should be developed for each new trial in which you participate, specific to the nuances of that trial.

Services not covered by Medicare include the following:

- Medical or hospital services related to the use of a device that the contractor decides are not "reasonable and necessary" for treatment of the Medicare beneficiary for whom you are seeking payment for their care while under the trial

- Medical and hospital services related to the use of a device that is excluded from coverage for other reasons (i.e., no benefit category or a national no coverage determination exists for the devices comparable to the study device)

Avoid billing pitfalls

Given the very particular requirements that must be met in order for Medicare to pay for use of a medical device under investigation, it is critical for health care professionals and providers of all types to ensure that they are submitting claims only for covered services.

First, you must know whether the device and the clinical trial, itself, are eligible for reimbursement. This is determined by how the FDA categorizes your device. You can only bill for Category B devices.

Be certain to request a copy of the FDA letter sent to the trial sponsor notifying the company as to whether its product is a Category A or a Category B device. All sponsors receive such a letter at the same time FDA notifies Medicare of the device categorization. A sponsor should not refuse or be reluctant to give this information to you. If the sponsor resists providing information about a device's categorization, do not agree to proceed with the clinical trial unless they relent, or if the sponsor agrees to pay for trial care, so you don't risk billing Medicare inappropriately.

Next, send the medical director of your Medicare contractor a package of the informational materials about the science and clinical efficacy of the investigational device and devices closely related to it.

Remember: Coverage is not automatic under the device regulation. The contractors must weigh the reasonableness and medical necessity of the device separately for each patient you enroll in the device clinical trial. Therefore, the investigator or investigational site should meet or speak with the FI or carrier charged with this decision before you enroll any participants, particularly if you think you are going to enroll large numbers of Medicare beneficiaries into the trial.

This meeting should familiarize the contractor with the investigational device and the clinical literature supporting its likely efficacy. Also get a sense of whether the contractor is inclined to pay for the device under trial. This could save you from being liable for the costs associated with the care of the patient enrolled in the trial. For example, if the carrier or FI decides against coverage, you and the sponsor have the opportunity initially to continue working with the medical director to show that coverage is justified. Alternatively, if the contractor seems quite sure the device will not be covered, the investigator can attempt to negotiate payment from the sponsor for the device and the related services. Again, this ensures that you will not be left having rendered services that will go unpaid.

If a contractor seems inclined toward coverage, request that the contractor put this opinion in writing for your records. It would not serve as a coverage decision for individual cases, but this written statement would provide at least some evidence that the carrier considers that the device may be appropriate for some individuals. A written opinion also shows that you tried to make a good faith effort to get the coverage and reimbursement right.

Audit billing for device trials regularly as part of your facility's broader compliance plan. These audits should verify that the patient's chart maintains all the necessary documentation about the study and the services furnished as part of the study, and that the only claims for services submitted for payment were those set forth in the protocol billing guidelines developed by the billing and clinical department.

If you maintain case reports to send the study results to the sponsors, ensure that the original documents indicating the services that trial participants received (and for which Medicare is being asked to reimburse) are in the medical record. Copies of the information may be placed in the case reports.

Patient-specific billing issues

As explained, contractors must determine coverage one patient at a time. This means each time you enroll a patient in a clinical trial for treatment with an investigational device, the claim submitted to the carrier or FI must put the contractor on notice that services furnished were related to the device and that the device is part of the trial. Each individual claim will also need to contain information that responds to the coverage criteria discussed earlier, unless the contractor agrees to use the packet of background materials you supplied before enrolling patients in the study as support for coverage for all claims submitted.

Contractors also take into consideration the setting in which the device was implanted or used to treat the trial participant, so make sure the site of service is appropriate. Base this decision on the level of difficulty and risk involved with the implantation or use of the investigational device and compare it to similar devices. It is also critical to remember that both the facility and the provider of the professional component services must identify claims related to a device trial.

Billing for devices under the NCD

In addition to the device regulation, devices are also eligible for coverage under the NCD, but only if they meet the specified criteria. Under the NCD, the cost of the experimental device would not be covered, but the routine costs associated with the device could be.

The NCD likely will cover more costs associated with the trial than the device coverage, but what method of coverage you pursue depends on what device you are testing. Generally, if the device itself is very expensive, and the sponsor is not paying for it, then it might make more sense to go through the device regulation, which pays for the cost of the device. If the device is less costly, it might be beneficial to seek coverage under the NCD.

Remember: You cannot use both sources of coverage. Choose one path, or risk violating fraud and abuse laws.

Device trials seeking reimbursement under the NCD must follow the same process as pharmaceutical trials, as outlined in the next section.

CHAPTER 3

The NCD Brings Changes for Trials

Chapter 3

The NCD Brings Changes for Trials

With the publication of the final NCD for clinical trials in 2000, CMS made its policy clear regarding Medicare coverage of the costs of routine health care services furnished to Medicare beneficiaries participating in certain clinical trials. The NCD makes it easier for providers to enroll subjects in clinical trials because subjects don't have to worry that their routine health care costs provided during a trial won't be paid.

What is an NCD?

An NCD is a national Medicare policy statement that identifies when the program will cover (pay for) particular items or services. NCDs affect beneficiaries nationwide, are prospective in nature, and describe the clinical circumstances and settings under which an item or service will be considered reasonable and necessary (or not). In some instances, Medicare uses the NCD to state that it no longer considers an item or service experimental or investigational. Once an NCD is issued, it is controlling, which means all Medicare contractors, including carriers, FIs, quality improvement organizations, health maintenance organizations, and Medicare+Choice organizations, are required to follow its mandate. Administrative law judges also must follow NCDs.

What is an NCD (cont.)

NCDs do not indicate what current procedural technology (CPT) code, if any, is assigned to a particular item or service determined to be covered.

If an item or service is not the subject of an NCD, or some type of program guidance found in Medicare manuals, local contractors can decide coverage and payment in the case of new items and services. These local policies, historically called local medical review policies (LMRPs), apply only to the suppliers and providers in the local contractor's jurisdiction.

An LMRP may contain any or all of the following: coding provisions, benefit category provisions, statutory exclusion provisions, and medical necessity provisions. Recently, Congress defined another type of decision that local contractors can make—local coverage determinations (LCDs). Although LCDs are similar to LMRPs, LCDs only pertain to decisions of medical necessity. In other words, they set the standard as to when a local contractor will consider an item or service reasonable and necessary. Like NCDs, LCDs do not say what CPT code to assign to a service or how much to pay providers for performing it.

Before an NCD goes into effect, CMS prepares claims processors for the change. The claims processors receive the following items in advance:

- Manual instruction
- Program memoranda
- CMS ruling
- *Federal Register* notice

What is an NCD? (cont.)

Along with directions regarding the NCD, CMS gives a date indicating when the NCD takes effect. In addition to providing instructions on the pending NCD, CMS also makes provisions to change billing and claims processing systems so payments can be processed. The NCD will then be published in the *Medicare Coverage Issues Manual*. It becomes effective the date it is published.

Source: CMS, www.cms.gov

At first glance, the NCD for clinical trials seems fairly straightforward. It says Medicare will cover the "routine costs" of "qualifying clinical trials," and items and services to treat complications from trial participation. It also states that all other Medicare rules apply to clinical trials as well. Yet despite the brevity of the provision and the uncomplicated language, ambiguities in the interpretation of several key words can make the coverage policy very difficult to apply.

The scope of the clinical trials coverage is determined through the definitions of the terms "routine costs" and "qualifying clinical trials." These two terms set forth what items or services Medicare will cover for beneficiaries participating in clinical trials.

Routine costs

Under the NCD, routine costs of a clinical trial include all items and services that otherwise would be generally available to Medicare beneficiaries regardless of whether they are assigned to the experimental or control arm of a clinical trial. "Generally available" means that the item or service falls within an existing Medicare benefit category (i.e., physician service), that it is not excluded from coverage by another provision in the law, and that is not the subject of an NCD stating that the item or service is not covered (i.e., acupuncture).

The following items and services are specifically included as a routine cost:

- Items or services typically provided absent a clinical trial (e.g., conventional care)

- Items or services required solely for the provision of the investigational item or service (e.g., administration of a noncovered chemotherapeutic agent)

- The clinically appropriate monitoring of the effects of the item or service, or the prevention of complications

- Items or services needed for reasonable and necessary care arising from the provision of an investigational item or service—in particular, for the diagnosis or treatment of complications

The following items and services are specifically excluded from the definition of routine cost:

- The investigational item or service, itself

- Items and services provided solely to satisfy data collection and analysis needs and that are not used in the direct clinical management of the patient (e.g., monthly computed tomography scans for a condition usually requiring only a single scan)

- Items and services customarily provided by the research sponsors free of charge for any enrollee in the trial

- Items and services provided solely to determine trial eligibility

For noncovered items and services, including items and services that federal law prohibits Medicare from paying for, the program only covers the treatment of complications arising from the delivery of the noncovered item or service and unrelated reasonable and necessary care.

> **Example:** Patient X is enrolled in a clinical trial designed to study a new laser for refractive eye surgery, which is considered cosmetic surgery. Medicare cannot pay for the procedure, and, therefore, the provider cannot submit claims under the NCD for any services related to the surgery, even if the services would otherwise be considered conventional care.

However, if a Medicare beneficiary in the clinical trial suffered a complication related to the surgery, however, Medicare would pay for any care furnished to the individual to treat the complication, provided Medicare would cover the treatment for patients not enrolled in a clinical trial.

You need the following two pieces of information to determine whether Medicare routinely covers an item or service, and, therefore, whether you can bill for it:

1. Whether the item or service falls into one of the four categories of routine costs noted above

2. Whether the item or service falls into any of the exclusion categories

This is one of the most difficult aspects of complying with the NCD.

Example: Patient X is admitted to the hospital to receive chemotherapy during the course of treatment for cancer. The chemotherapy is under investigation as part of a clinical trial considered to be a qualified trial. The standard of care requires that patients who receive chemotherapy be observed for complications during the infusion, and that they have certain tests performed to monitor for adverse side effects. The protocol also requires patient X to undergo an echocardiogram to document that the chemotherapy is not weakening his heart.

Without some type of statement from Medicare that the hospital observation or laboratory work is not covered, or without evidence that sponsors customarily paid for these services prior to the NCD, the hospital should be able to bill Medicare for these services. However, the hospital could not bill Medicare for the drug under investigation. Medicare also should not be billed for the echocardiogram if the procedure would not be considered part of the conventional care of patients. This would be the case if the echocardiogram is not part of Patient X's treatment, but is used solely to document a particular aspect of the safety profile of the drug.

Qualifying clinical trials

Mandatory qualifying criteria

If providers want Medicare to consider any items and services eligible for reimbursement under the NCD, they must provide them within a certain category of clinical trials, referred to as "qualified clinical trials." The trial must be designed to evaluate an item or service that falls within a Medicare benefit category (e.g., physicians' service, durable medical equipment, diagnostic test) and that is not statutorily excluded from coverage (e.g., cosmetic surgery, hearing aids). The trial also may not be designed only to test toxicity or disease pathophysiology. In other words, the study must have therapeutic intent. And finally, unless the trial is designed to study a diagnostic intervention, the inclusion criteria of the protocol must require that participants be individuals with diagnosed disease rather than healthy volunteers. Trials involving diagnostic intervention may enroll healthy patients in order to have a proper control group.

In addition to the three mandatory criteria above, a clinical trial also must have certain other desirable characteristics in order for routine costs to be covered by Medicare. To ensure that reimbursement is given to trials with these characteristics, the NCD requires that a clinical trial either be *deemed* to have these characteristics or be *certified* as having them.

Desirable characteristics

The required desirable characteristics are as follows:

- The principal purpose of the trial is to test whether the intervention potentially improves the participants' health outcomes

- The trial is well-supported by available scientific and medical information, or it is intended to clarify or establish the health outcomes of interventions already in common clinical use

- It does not unjustifiably duplicate existing studies

- The trial design is appropriate to answer the research question being posed in the trial

• The trial is sponsored by a credible organization or individual capable of executing the proposed trial successfully

• The trial complies with federal regulations relating to the protection of human subjects

• All aspects of the trial are conducted according to the appropriate standards of scientific integrity

The qualification and enrollment process

Principal investigators are required by the NCD to certify that the trial meets mandatory qualifying criteria and has the desirable characteristics. They must also enroll the trial with CMS. Because determining whether a trial has the desirable characteristics is particularly subjective, CMS set forth two mechanisms to guide this decision.

First, a trial will be **"deemed"** to have the desirable characteristics if it is conducted with oversight by a federal agency or authority. Trials in this category include the following:

• Trials funded or supported by centers of cooperative groups that are funded by NIH, Centers for Disease Control and Prevention (CDC), the Agency for Healthcare Research and Quality (AHRQ), CMS, Department of Defense (DOD), and Department of Veterans Affairs (VA)

- Trials conducted under an investigational new drug application (IND) reviewed by the FDA

- Drug trials exempt from having IND (under 21 CFR 312.2(b)(1)) are automatically qualified until qualifying criteria are developed and the certification process is in place.

Principal investigators of deemed trials do not have to certify that the study meets the desirable characteristics; they only have to enroll the trial in the Medicare clinical trials registry. However, the registry has not yet been established. Consequently, until the registry becomes available, sponsors of IND trials and IND-exempt trials are expected to notify Medicare of any trial under which routine cost coverage may be sought. A sponsor accomplishes this by sending an e-mail to *clinicaltrials@cms.hhs.gov*.

If a trial does not qualify for deemed status, then principal investigators must **certify** that their study has the desirable characteristics.

To ensure some level of consistency across certified trials, the proposed NCD protocol states that the AHRQ will convene a multi-agency panel comprised of representatives from the Department of Health and Human Services (HHS) research agencies (NIH, CDC, FDA, AHRQ, and the Office of Human Research Protection), and the research arms of the DOD and the VA to develop a set of criteria that, if met, would be a strong indication that a trial had the desirable characteristics.

These criteria are supposed to be easily verifiable so it will be relatively easy for a principal investigator to determine whether his or her study has the necessary desirable characteristics needed for coverage. This panel cannot review or approve individual trials. Its purpose is solely to develop the criteria and to meet periodically thereafter to review and evaluate the program and recommend any necessary refinements to CMS.

This set of criteria has yet to be issued, so there is currently no mechanism in place to qualify a trial for NCD coverage unless it is a deemed study. This likely reflects the mixed feelings within HHS and the life sciences industry itself about the availability of coverage for trials not under any oversight by the federal government. There is an argument that private research tends to reflect private interests, that it may be biased in its design and therefore should not be supported by government funds. Yet not all government-sponsored research is above speculation of conflicts of interest.

The real issue, however, is whether the government ever plans to establish qualifying criteria that would allow private research to receive reimbursement. The need for clinical research is increasing as companies push products and services to commercialization quicker. Nevertheless, not all pharmaceutical companies support the push for this process to begin. In some ways it may actually benefit these companies to keep things they way they are today. Companies working through trials under federal oversight enjoy the benefit of deemed status and coverage for many of the costs related to trials for their new products. As a result, participant recruitment for these trials should, at least theoretically, be easier.

CHAPTER 4

Negotiating with Sponsors

Chapter 4

Negotiating with Sponsors

One of the trickiest and most overwhelming aspects of being a clinical trials investigator is negotiating the payment and terms of the project with the sponsor. As an independent contractor, you have little leverage. However, this is starting to change as investigators and sites are becoming more sophisticated in their dealings with sponsors, and as sponsor-investigator relationships have come under the microscope of government enforcement agencies. This scrutiny is expected to become more intense because of the NCD and the fact that Medicare dollars are now in play.

The research agreement: Get it in writing

Before you start any type of clinical research project, have an agreement in place to ensure that the costs involved with the trial are reimbursed and to describe the relationship between the investigator and the sponsor. To decrease business and legal risk, this agreement must be captured in a contract signed by both parties before the investigator enrolls any participants into the trial.

Generally a clinical trials agreement should

- define the scope of the work expected of the investigator

- establish acceptable payment arrangements

- address important issues such as protection of confidential information, compliance with the Health Insurance Portability and Accountability Act of 1996 privacy and security standards

- liability insurance and indemnification in the event of third-party injury

- ownership of any data generated

- the right to publish research results, and the ownership of intellectual property or the right to develop intellectual property

The contract also should specify that investigator is an independent contractor and include a provision that addresses termination of the study. Investigators in particular should demand that the contract clearly state the financial responsibility of the sponsor with respect to costs accrued by the investigator if the sponsor terminates the contract early.

Negotiating the terms

Before entering into negotiations with a sponsor, read the research protocol thoroughly to understand the scope of the work and the expense involved and to determine whether you can carry it out successfully. Analyze all the costs involved to decide whether the payment from the sponsor is fair-market value.

Some, but not all, of the questions you need to answer include the following:

- Is your staff willing and able to take on the extra work of the clinical trial? Will you have to hire additional personnel to fulfill the administrative and clinical requirements of the protocol?

- Does your staff have the skill needed to carry out the protocol?

- How many procedures, labs, diagnostic tests and follow-up visits are required, and of what intensity?

- Will Medicare or any other payer cover the costs of any of the items or services you will provide to trial participants?

- What is the length of trial?

- What is the time commitment of patients?

- What clinical supplies are needed? Will you have to stock supplies beyond those you generally keep?

- What are the potential risks and benefits of the trial? Are the risks reasonable? What is the potential harm to your reputation among the remainder of your patients and the community if there is a bad outcome related to the trial?

- Is there a minimum number of patients you are expected to enroll? Will you be able to achieve this goal and maintain the integrity of the inclusion/exclusion criteria?

- How will data collection be documented and maintained?

- What work will be needed to close out your participation in the trial?

After considering the issue above, **prepare a working budget.** The budget protects you from being over- or underpaid. Include start-up costs, time, and resources required to meet the elements of the protocol. These include costs related to screening, even if the participant is not enrolled in the study or does not complete the protocol, and any additional obligations, such as travel to investigator's meetings and training your staff on the details of the study. In addition, develop a second-draft budget that addresses potential unanticipated costs, such as unscheduled patient visits, lab mistakes requiring repeat testing, or treatment for adverse events.

Payment terms

The three types of research agreements are generally characterized based on the method of payment to the investigator or investigative site. The first type of agreement is a **cost-reimbursement agreement.** This contract obligates a sponsor to pay for actual costs incurred by the investigator up to a maximum amount. The next type of agreement is a **fixed-priced contract** that obligates the sponsor to pay the investigator an agreed-upon flat fee for services. The final type of agreement is the **flat-rate contract** that specifies an agreed-upon amount per unit of service. Flat-rate contracts generally are based on a click fee per participant enrolled in the study.

To decrease your legal risk and the risk of billing Medicare inappropriately, pay close attention to the payment schedule of a clinical trials agreement. Any payment received should be fair-market value for services rendered by the investigator and for expenses incurred.

Traditionally, most clinical trial contracts have been either fixed-price or flat rate. Both types provide the sponsor and investigator the greatest flexibility in determining a payment rate. Each minimizes the transactions costs for sponsors, particularly when they are negotiating with less sophisticated parties who are unlikely to question the breakdown of non-itemized payments. Lump-sum contracts have also provided sponsors with some cover to counter kickback allegations, since nonspecific payment amounts provide greater flexibility to argue about fair-market value for services. Nevertheless, such lump-sum payments without any explanation of the services they are meant to cover can put researchers and sponsors at risk for allegations of false claims if the researchers intend to bill Medicare for any items or services rendered in connection with the clinical trial.

Improper billing

There is much uncertainty about what is covered or not covered under Medicare. The NCD provides clearer direction than many other regulations or statements by CMS, but there are still some twists and turns that complicate the process. Obviously, you can't submit claims to Medicare for items or services paid for by the sponsor. Yet, without a sufficient breakdown of the payments from a sponsor, trial administrators could receive money from the government to which they are not entitled. At a minimum, you would have to refund this money to Medicare.

These overpayments also could lead to allegations by the government that the claim was false, and potentially subject the researcher and trial site to a False Claims Act investigation. Depending on the circumstances surrounding the matter, the government also could pursue action against the sponsor for conspiracy to submit false claims if it can show that the sponsor knew that the claims were being submitted to Medicare inappropriately. Though a more tenuous legal theory, the government also could try to develop a conspiracy argument against a sponsor who intentionally avoided entering into contracts with itemized payment schedules so clinicians would have greater flexibility in their billing options.

Another area of potential risk associated with billing involves submitting claims to Medicare for items traditionally paid for by the sponsor. By including this provision, in the regulations CMS put the industry on notice that it would be watching for trends suggesting sponsors were trying to shift research costs they traditionally incurred to the Medicare program. The problem with this provision, however, is that it is very difficult to determine what is "traditional" in sponsor contracts, particularly if your facility is not an established research site.

Investigators should seek assurances from sponsors that the items and services that they're paying for are things they have commonly paid for in the past. If the sponsors won't offer these assurances, ask them to pay for the items and services that would have been billed to Medicare, because you would be unable to do so under the contract.

Beware of confidentiality agreements

Sponsor agreements often have a confidentiality clause, which can limit trial administrators from releasing information. That clause can prevent clinicians from releasing information to the payer. Be certain to either negotiate with sponsors to remove this provision, or see whether they will allow you to submit a summary version of the protocol to the payer.

CHAPTER 5

Billing Private Insurers

Chapter 5

Billing Private Insurers

As complicated as it may be to bill Medicare for trial-related costs, billing private insurance companies can be much more difficult—if you can get them to pay at all. Most don't. In many ways, the situation with respect to private payers resembles the situation under Medicare before the federal program began supplying some coverage under device and NCD rules. Most private payers only cover medically necessary items or services "unrelated" to an investigational item or service, just as Medicare used to do. If a private payer does offer some coverage for clinical research–related items or services, it will likely be only for what Medicare would call "routine" services—items related to the investigational device or treatment, but not the device or treatment itself.

What's covered: A moving target

One of the most challenging aspects of billing private payers is trying to determine what, if anything, they cover. Some provider agreements contain a statement that excludes investigational items or services and anything related from coverage. These provisions are disappointing in their lack of any commitment to clinical research. But at least they are reasonably clear on the basic issue of coverage, despite the fact that they don't help you distinguish "related" or "unrelated" services or items.

Most payers consider conventional care related to a complication from a clinical research trial to be unrelated to the trial for purposes of determining coverage. But the dividing line between "related" and "unrelated" is often unclear. In a frustrating number of cases, this line is also a moving target, with private payers seeming to make a series of inconsistent determinations in similar and, sometimes, factually indistinguishable situations.

Research institutions, investigators, billing managers, and research coordinators all complain about a lack of clarity that extends beyond the issue of what is related or unrelated to clinical research. The question of what coverage a private payer offers beyond unrelated items and services is frequently less than clear. A review of many provider agreements will reveal their restrictions using very ambiguous language. For example, you might see a statement indicating that "only medically necessary services are covered." This leaves participants in clinical research guessing whether particular items or services related to a trial might be covered.

Cutting through the confusion

The following steps can help the participants in clinical research sort through the confusing situation they will routinely face when determining whether a private payer will cover any costs connected to a clinical trial.

However, we should start with a basic observation about timing: It is critically important to undertake the process of clarifying what a private payer will and will not pay for as early as possible in the process. It's preferable that you start this process before your research institution even signs its agreement with the sponsoring organization.

The reason for this is quite simple: It will help your organization determine what private and governmental sources will be providing support for the trial under the contract terms for clinical research–related items or services. Without that information, you may waste the sponsoring organization's support, as private payers typically will have coordination clauses in their provider agreements. These clauses stipulate that, even where the payer would normally provide payment, the payer is relieved from that responsibility because the costs at issue have already been reimbursed.

Another important reason to determine what is covered is that this information is critically important in deciding whether to conduct the research. All too often, institutions make long-term contractual commitments to undertake research based on assumptions about the collateral sources of available financial support. These assumptions often prove less than accurate. Such a failure may turn a potential financial benefit into a financial disaster, or at least a financial disappointment.

Early consideration of these issues is also important because the process can be a long one. It becomes more complicated once the clinical trial has begun and the opportunity to proceed in an ordered, proactive manner is lost. So determine coverage **before** the trial begins, not after you have already enrolled subjects and the research is underway.

Some institutions and their busy research coordinators and billing managers put off clarifying coverage. They are pressed by other assignments, and they believe, incorrectly, that the process cannot start until the subjects are enrolled and their insurance status is determined. There is no need to delay, because, depending on the enrollment criteria, it is a virtual certainty that you will be dealing with most of the major payers in the marketplace during the trial. You might as well start with those payers.

Five steps to determining coverage

Step 1: Begin by finding out whether a third party has already started determining coverage for you and your institution. Often, sponsors will have collected information on major insurance plans, as may other research sites involved in the research your institution is considering to pursue. This is one of the many advantages of being involved in multi-site research. Also, determine whether someone within your own organization—the billing manager or the research coordinator for a previous study—may have collected the necessary information.

With that said, however, use care when relying upon information from third parties. Verify the accuracy and completeness of any information supplied by a third party. Regrettably, there are many instances of research sites that discuss these issues with other outside research sites, sponsoring organizations, or other third parties and learn later, to their regret, that the information was less than accurate.

If you cannot find the information you are looking for from the research sponsor or other third parties, consider the following steps:

Step 2: Write the insurance company and ask whether it has a policy on trial-related coverage. You might receive a response with a reasonably helpful policy enclosed. You might receive a letter that restates some or all of the applicable clauses from the research site's provider agreement with the payer and gives some additional guidance by way of some interpretative gloss on those clauses. You may receive nothing. Unfortunately, many companies will not have a written policy on this topic. Even if you do not receive much —if anything—helpful in response to your request, it is important to send a written request. A documented effort to secure this kind of written guidance can be very helpful in the event of a dispute at some later date between the insurer and your institution regarding coverage and the clarity of the payer's policy.

Step 3: Contact someone within the coverage, payment, or contracting offices of the insurance company and ask for information on coverage. Start by calling the medical director, a coverage review specialist (who is typically someone with a nursing background), or special operations people within the coverage or even the payment review units.

Be aware that this process may take some time and cause some frustration. Not only is it difficult to track down the information you are looking for, but insurance companies may often refer you to different personnel to address their various insurance products, which may all provide slightly different coverages and coverage limitations.

Step 4: Go to the subject's employer for help. Do not forget that the insurance company's customer typically is the employer who selected that coverage for its employees and who is paying the lion's share of the health care costs associated with the insurance. Indeed, in many instances, an insurance company may simply be serving as a third party administrator of the employer's own self-funded program. In situations such as this, refer your coverage questions to the subject's employer to discuss coverage options, or you may be able to exert additional pressure on the insurance company by involving the employer. This may be time-consuming, but you might find that approaching the employer helps secure some coverage in cases where it would not otherwise be available.

Step 5: In arguing for coverage with a private payer, think about other allies to bring into the debate, besides the subject's employer. Consider the following potential allies in these situations:

- Patient advocacy groups

- State legislators

- State insurance commissions or state departments of insurance or managed care

Emphasizing the absence of any alternative treatment for the condition being studied can be an effective argument in attempting to secure assistance from groups and offices such as these.

State insurance commissions and departments of managed care can help, but only if they have jurisdiction over the plan at issue. So confirm that the plan at issue is subject to the regulatory control of the agency you have contacted before beginning to work with that department on the issue.

State insurance commissions and departments of managed care and insurance can provide assistance on these sort of insurance coverage issues because of their broad regulatory oversight powers, and because plans are regularly required by state law to file a statement outlining what costs they will and will not cover. By denying a particular claim for payment based on an ambiguous restriction, an insurance company might be seen as acting in a manner inconsistent with its filing. State agencies have a duty to ensure that plans under their jurisdiction deliver the coverage they say they will provide. If the agency makes an inquiry and expresses concern, a payer may well conclude that it should reverse its earlier determination. Even small penalties, when imposed by an insurance regulator, can have significant public relations and other implications for a payer.

Relying on the guidance you've secured

In any situation in which you secure coverage or reimbursement and you intend to rely upon that information, document the advice you received in the event of a dispute. If the payer does not put its guidance in writing to you and your institution, write to the payer contact who was the source of the information, restate the question you posed, list the information provided to you in response, and state your intention to rely on the information provided to you, unless informed in writing within a limited time-period that the guidance was incorrect or requires modification.

Some payers may deny they have received such confirmation letters after disputes arise between research sites and the payers. Consider sending these confirmation letters by certified or overnight mail so there is documentation of their delivery. Also, make sure to save these sorts of confirmation letters in a single, readily accessible place in the event of a dispute. All too often, this sort of valuable evidence of the good faith efforts of research sites to understand and follow coverage restrictions winds up in an individual patient's billing, accounts receivable, or medical records, where it is essentially unretrievable in the event of any dispute not focused on that patient.

However, as a formal matter, this type of confirmation might not be legally binding on the payer. Agreements with private payers likely state that the contract language is binding unless a written modification has been signed. Notwithstanding that possible argument, a confirmation letter should at least demonstrate that you acted in good faith, and that any incorrect claims you submitted based on any inaccurate information you received do not constitute fraud or abuse. As a practical matter, if not a legal one, the presence of a confirmation letter will make it difficult for payers to enforce a contrary position.

Possible fraud and abuse issues

Unfortunately, some research institutions and organizations believe (quite incorrectly) that they need not be as precise and as focused in their private-payer compliance efforts as they are with federally funded health care programs. This is a dangerous misconception, because both the federal and state governments have a variety of means to target claims filed for noncovered items or services related to clinical research trials. State laws typically make "insurance fraud" a punishable offense, and many states now have state false claims acts patterned on the federal False Claims Act that apply to claims filed with private health care payers. The federal government also has ample means to address issues involving private payers. For example, the "all plan" health care fraud provision enacted as part of HIPAA makes it a federal crime to engage in fraud involving either a public or a private plan. Basic criminal statutes such as mail and wire fraud prohibitions can be powerful vehicles for the federal government to investigate and punish fraudulent conduct involving private payers.

A final note about private pay coverage

If investigated properly, reimbursements from private insurers may benefit your organization's research efforts. The sponsor and government payers are two pieces of the financial puzzle when examining the financial impact of participation in a study. But as noted earlier, private payers may also be relevant and could offer a third source of reimbursement.

CHAPTER 6

Continuous Compliance Improvement

Chapter 6

Continuous Compliance Improvement

Problems come in many forms

In October 2003, the Department of Justice (DOJ) reached settlements with seven hospitals for improperly billing Medicare for experimental cardiac devices. The settlement amounts ranged from $115,000 to $3.2 million. These settlements brought the total price of DOJ settlements for false billing of cardiac devices to $40 million. All of these settlements related to a whistleblower False Claims Act case, initiated by a salesman turned whistleblower, who reported a number of hospitals for improperly billing for the devices he was selling them. The hospitals were allegedly billing both Medicare and TRICARE for the experimental defibrillator and related services. To date, this has been the most high-profile case in which the government has cracked down on false claims relating to experimental devices. But there have been others.

For example, consider a case that targeted the University of Minnesota. It involved allegations that the university had, for more than two decades, billed for an experimental drug that had not yet received FDA approval.

While the actual loss to the federal government was tallied at some $85 million, the government recognized the value of the research performed at the university and settled for a "mere" $32 million. It agreed to accept that amount not entirely in cash, but also through the creation of a university-funded $24 million in additional research. This allowed the NIH to reduce funding it would otherwise have likely supplied.

In addition to the above cases, the government also investigated several institutions (mostly before the NCD) that were alleged to have applied the "related to" criteria inappropriately in an attempt to have Medicare pay clinical research-related costs.

Even after the NCD was issued, these types of problems continue in connection with research that does not qualify for coverage under the NCD.

Given the complexities of billing for clinical trials, you or your institution may encounter problems related to clinical trials coverage or billing issues. Some who have been involved in clinical trials research for many years might even tell you that confronting a crisis or two is inevitable.

For example, sometimes an organization might not consider an item or service to be experimental even though the government does—i.e., the off-label use of medications. A drug itself may be FDA approved, but the off-label use may be considered experimental by the government, even though your organization might have concluded differently.

Facing problems

Trouble, unfortunately, can come in many forms, including any of the
following:

- An audit letter from Medicare

- A subpoena under the HIPAA All Plan fraud provision, which makes
  it a violation of criminal law to commit various acts of fraud on any
  health care plan, including private plans

- A grand jury subpoena

- A letter from the DOJ notifying your organization that a whistleblower action has been filed

- A piece of correspondence from a private insurance company alleging
  insurance fraud related to clinical trials billing

- A call from a reporter with the local paper, regarding an internal memorandum that the paper has obtained, discussing whether clinical trial–
  related services have been billed incorrectly to the Medicare program

- An employee calls the compliance officer and raises an issue related to
  improper clinical trial billing

Establishing a proactive system

If any of these or similar issues arise, you need a solid plan to deal with them. If you have to design a process to respond to the issue when it occurs, then your response will be inadequate, and you will wish that you had responded more proactively. Part of responding proactively means establishing well thought-out billing systems to process claims effectively while preventing fraud issues from materializing in the first place. Even well-designed systems cannot avert every problem, so it is also important to develop procedures to monitor your system and manage problems as they arise.

Establishing an effective claims-processing system

There are many ways to make sure that claims submitted to the government are timely, complete, and accurate. The key to the success of any system is consistency and continuous monitoring.

The billing process begins when you ask a sponsor if you can serve as an investigator or your facility can serve as an investigative site for a trial. At this point, the investigator receives information about the protocol and the work that will be expected of him or her. In many instances, the sponsor also will provide initial information on compensation for serving as an investigator.

Sponsors often pressure investigators to decide quickly whether to serve as an investigator. Depending on the competition for various research projects, sponsors may simply move on to the next interested party if your response is delayed. At the same time, potential investigators must examine the sponsor proposal carefully and analyze the cost of the project before agreeing to participate. Pay particular attention to what items and services the sponsor intends to cover, and what items it will not.

As discussed earlier, sponsor proposals are best vetted when the potential investigator, his or her clinical trials coordinator, and a member of the billing or insurance staff decide whether Medicare or another payer would cover the items and services the sponsor won't cover. The investigator should list the items and services believed to be routine care, and what items and services will be performed strictly to fulfill the protocol. Once this list is completed, a member of the billing staff should list items likely to be reimbursed and items likely not to be reimbursed. If any ambiguity exists as to the coverage of any item, the billing expert should contact the FI or carrier for guidance. This is particularly true when the trial involves an investigational device. The contractor can decide whether to cover a trial at all, not just what items or services will be allowed, as is the case with the NCD.

This process ensures that the clinical and billing staff understand what may be billed to Medicare and other payers. It also provides the investigator with an assessment of the cost of the trial, so he or she may try to negotiate payment adjustments with the sponsor, if necessary. If a gap appears between what the sponsor will to pay for and what Medicare or other payers will cover, the investigator must be willing to accept the remaining financial risk of participating.

Once the trial is underway, the routine-items list can serve as a template for a charge ticket. The provider furnishing a service payable under the NCD simply circles the item or service on the charge ticket to indicate that it was performed, and the billing staff can be confident that the item or service may billed under the NCD, since the investigator determined previously what he or she considers to be routine care.

Your computer systems also can prevent research claims from slipping through the cracks by setting internal commands to flag clinical trials claims for hand review. Your system could also be programmed with the start and end dates for trials so claims outside of this window are not processed. Beware of computer systems that automatically try to match services with covered diagnosis codes. If the code identified does not match the reason why the procedure was performed, it could cause problems.

In addition to using mechanisms to identify research-related claims, also ensure that your staff can process them. It may help to identify one person to handle research claims. This person should be involved in all discussions with clinical coordinators and other meetings in regard to any particular protocol. If an outside vendor does your billing, the clinical trials coordinator and the billing staff member involved with the protocol should meet with a vendor representative to create a method to ensure that the billing company knows about claims related to trials—both device trials and NCD trials.

Most important in protecting yourself from the risk of receiving overpayments or incurring potential false claims liability is to ensure that you have an effective compliance program and that research issues are an integral part of that program. If you already have a program, augment it with standards of conduct for research issues, as well as policies and procedures putting these standards into practice. In addition, include in any audit protocol a benchmark for claims and medical record documentation of services furnished in a trial, regardless of whether it's an IDE trial or and NCD trial.

Building a strong compliance program

The foundation of any solid billing program is a solid compliance program. Clinical trials possess a number of complexities and unique qualities, including billing and coverage issues. For this reason, it may be wise to separate the clinical trials compliance program from your general compliance program. Simply adding clinical research trials issues to a general compliance program reduces the chance that they will get the attention they deserve.

Your compliance program can be entirely separate from your traditional compliance program, or it can be loosely connected with the main program. Often the best solution is to have the clinical research program operate as a module, or subcomponent, of the overall program. Remember to address all critical issues separately under easy-to-access headings.

Draft standards for all

You must draft your standards on clinical trials issues for a very broad audience with entirely distinct experiences, perspectives, and outlooks. Make them useful and instructive to researchers, research coordinators, billing managers, coders, technologists, nurses, and a host of others involved in clinical research.

Some institutions elect to keep their standards quite general, leaving the details of compliance for a separate set of policies. That approach may permit a more tailored discussion of issues. However, some institutions, particularly community hospitals and regional medical centers involved in research, take an "all or nothing" approach to these general standards. They either deal with all of the critical issues in detail in their standards, or never get around to addressing them.

Experience is key

When deciding how to structure your program, keep in mind that clinical trials billing issues are unique and distinct, as are compliance standards. Very competent hospital compliance officers may have almost no exposure to clinical trials. For that reason, they may not be well positioned to deal with billing issues—particularly in a crisis situation. Knowledge about clinical research is a must in directing, managing, and operating a successful program.

Accordingly, a current or former research study coordinator might be the perfect person to handle clinical trials billing issues as they arise. Such a candidate may need to receive some significant initial instruction regarding research coverage and billing issues in order to be effective in these areas, as even an experienced research study coordinator may have relatively little experience with the arcane issues discussed in this text. With smaller research programs, someone working part-time could be compliance officer or coordinator for clinical research issues. However, it is important to ensure that any part-time assistance does not pose a conflict of interest that would undermine the integrity of the program, or tarnish its image.

Share the responsibility

It is also important to emphasize that more than one person can oversee clinical trials compliance. A committee can perform the compliance function. In fact, for some involved in research compliance, it is critical to assign the oversight function to a committee in order to bring a wealth of different perspectives to the management of the program. An effective committee can consist of people within the institution's research community. For the purpose of addressing coverage and billing issues, this can include an investigator, a research coordinator, the billing manager, and a coder.

Still, even with a dedicated clinical research compliance committee, you need the kind of direction, focus, and accountability that can only come from appointing a single person as the primary overseer for clinical research compliance. Whether that person is dubbed a research compliance officer or coordinator, pick a single person to coordinate the committee's efforts to ensure that it has adequate resources at its disposal and that those resources are arrayed appropriately. He or she should also ensure that those who are delegated tasks are undertaking their responsibilities in an effective and timely fashion and that the organization responds quickly but carefully in a crisis.

Make training specific and ongoing

As the first step toward establishing a solid program, ensure that the relevant staff members understand clinical trials–related billing and coverage. Compliance training on general reimbursement and coverage issues helps only marginally in meeting this goal, given the unique issues raised by clinical research trials. Lecture-style sessions describing the rules that apply in clinical research—the NCD, the device coverage provision, etc.—help lay a foundation for the required competency.

However, experience teaches that the most effective means of education is specific training focused on the reimbursement implications of each element of research protocols before they are implemented.

Education sessions directed at the differing needs of the various participants in clinical research who need coverage and reimbursement information (including investigators, research coordinators, clinical department managers, billers, etc.) will ensure that training is relevant and meaningful. Many institutions, particularly smaller facilities, tend to see training on research compliance as a "one-shot deal." Repetition is often the best teacher in areas as complex as the coverage and reimbursement rules for clinical research trials.

Auditing and monitoring

The second element of an effective compliance program is auditing and monitoring programs. It is not enough to train personnel on clinical trials compliance; you need monitoring and auditing to confirm that the training has worked.

Monitoring and auditing can and should take many forms. Start by auditing samples of services and their underlying documentation. With presubmission audits, you may identify problems before you receive overpayments that need to be refunded. Post-payment audits offer no similar benefit. But even a presubmission audit will frequently yield results that will compel a disclosure or a repayment of an overpayment you received before the audit began. Make sure that the samples being reviewed reflect a cross-section of services billed.

Often smaller, more frequent audits work better than infrequent but comprehensive audits. In other words, if an institution insists upon very large samples before conducting an audit, it will likely find that it can only audit infrequently. Even busy compliance auditors and officers can conduct more focused audits more often, perhaps as frequently as monthly or quarterly. Generally speaking, the more frequent the audits, the more effectively they will identify issues early and keep research personnel focused on compliance as a critical issue.

We strongly recommend that a third-party auditor validate and supplement the findings of internal auditors at least every two years, and preferably every year. Auditors are often only as effective as the assumptions and the perspective that they bring to their audits. External auditors bring the benefit of possibly different assumptions and a more detached perspective.

Other forms of monitoring can also be extremely effective. In one helpful component of an effective monitoring program, personnel involved in research must complete compliance surveys that ask them to identify compliance issues, among others things. Selected interviews of a range of different personnel with a range of experience and perspectives are also helpful. Though time-consuming, interviews have the advantage of being more in-depth than written surveys; they also can be an important vehicle for the institution to express its commitment to compliance in a direct and personal fashion. Interviews can also can limit whistleblower activity because research personnel can clearly convey through these interviews the message that the institution will "do the right thing," if given an opportunity to do so. Finally, another valuable tool is a "walkthrough," in which compliance personnel take the role of a patient and get a first-hand view, in a hypothetical experience, of how a service is documented and billed.

Establish key relationships with outside experts

When it comes to dealing with a difficult challenge under clinical trial coverage and reimbursement rules, it also is critical to know where you can obtain accurate information and advice when needed. For this reason, it is very important to establish a relationship with outside counsel, a reimbursement consultant and auditor, and other key advisors.

Take care selecting experts in clinical research coverage and reimbursement. There are many health care and compliance experts out there, but expertise in nursing home compliance or the billing of nursing home stays, for example, won't help with clinical research.

Expert assistance can help in several ways, including the following:

- Training

- Auditing and monitoring

- Developing billing strategies based on the research protocol

- Drafting or reviewing compliance policies or billing instruction sheets

- Creating documentation guides and templates

- Responding to audit letters and subpoenas

- Answering press inquiries about an investigation

Depending on the resources of the research institution, use experts when you need the perspective gained from wide experience, when the demands of a tight deadline give little time for action, or when objectivity is needed to be effective or to bring credibility to a task. Invest some time early in the relationship with key advisors to give them a sense of the big picture so they are reasonably knowledgeable about your systems, organizational structure, personnel, compliance program and policies, and other basic information. This will make your experts more effective and more efficient in their work, giving you the benefit of lower-cost, high-quality services. Further, this kind of context can be essential in responding quickly and appropriately in crises posed by such challenges as a press inquiry or a search warrant.

Create policies and systems to deal with crises

As noted above, if you only start to think about how to respond to a challenge once it presents itself, your institution and your program are not likely to avoid or limit damage. Have a policy that deals with each of the following:

- Press inquiries

- Audit or overpayment demand letters

- Subpoenas

- Search warrants

A central component of all of these policies is ensuring that personnel are instructed to direct relevant issues immediately to a centralized contact trained to deal with these challenges. That central contact may either be an internal or external expert, though provision of external expertise is absolutely essential, at some point, with these types of issues. Many institutions do not have written policies to deal with these challenges. Those that do often have provided little or no training on these policies. Provide significant and repeated training on these policies to ensure that when staff are involved in a crisis, they will comply with them.

Although the contents of each of these policies will vary, depending upon the subject to be addressed and your program's structure, culture, and needs, the following are some elements that should be considered for many, if not all of them:

- The triggering event for the policy

- Who should be notified and how

- Who will coordinate the response

- How to store and protect pertinent documents

- Who will protect relevant documents

- When and how to coordinate with other departments, advisors, or others who will need to be updated and consulted

- Instructions on how to preserve the attorney-client privilege appropriately (which will include educating employees on how this protection works, what information is protected, and what is not protected)

- Ensuring that responsive documents are date- and number-stamped as a means of document control

Another critical policy should discuss document retention and destruction, and the appropriate mechanism by which to edit or add to existing clinical, billing, and other pertinent records. It is critical to ensure that these policies reflect the requirements of applicable federal and state law, including those imposed by the HIPAA, which made it a federal crime to engage in fraud involving either a public or private health plan.

Though almost a cliché, it is nevertheless true that many crises are heavily influenced by appropriate document management, a subject discussed in greater detail below. There is nothing as self-destructive or damning as documents that are destroyed or altered in response to a press inquiry, a subpoena, or a search warrant, or in anticipation of such an event. Accordingly, your policies should include a clear and unambiguous directive that if a subpoena or other legal process is reasonably likely, then any planned destruction of related documents will automatically be halted.

Create a culture that fosters compliance

Attitudes can help shape how people respond in a crisis and whether their conduct in the normal course of the day creates the seeds of crisis. Depending on the culture of an organization and the depth of its commitment to ethics—not just legalisms—program personnel can either respond to a situation in a narrow, legalistic effort to cover themselves, or they can view the crisis as a challenge to be overcome by acting in a principled and ethical manner. Organizations should also ensure their employees know that compliance is not only required, but also that following rules is about doing the right thing—about being ethical.

CHAPTER 7

Frequently Asked Questions

Chapter 7

Frequently Asked Questions

Billing Medicare for trial-related services can be complicated. The following is a sampling of commonly asked questions. We hope the answers will help you sort through issues that you might encounter.

Q **The research budget for my trial covers procedure costs, lab costs, etc. If the physician's standard practice includes an electrocardiogram, which is also required by the study, can I bill this to Medicare?**

A Medicare covers routine clinical trials costs, including all items and services for beneficiaries in the control or the experimental arm of a qualifying study. Assuming that your study is a qualifying study, routine services include "items or services that are typically provided absent a clinical trial (e.g., medically necessary conventional care")" for which there is a Medicare benefit category, and which are not subject to a Medicare non-coverage policy. Absent another Medicare policy that would not permit payment for the electrocardiogram, it should be covered.

Keep in mind, however, that providers cannot "double dip." If the research budget includes payment for a necessary service that is also considered routine care—and the clinical trial sponsor is paying for it—it cannot be billed to Medicare. In addition, if the sponsor would customarily pay for the service, Medicare will not cover it.

 Do you use the V70.7 diagnosis code on any Medicare claims for IDE device trials?

No. Under the IDE benefit, carriers must determine medical necessity for each beneficiary. Therefore, alert carriers that a claim involves payment in relation to an investigational Category B device. Do this by using the QA modifier and inserting the IDE number assigned to the device in item 23 field of the HCFA-1500. For electronic claims, the device number is entered in the DAO field. In addition, providers should consider providing a copy of the IDE approval letter to substantiate the claim for payment.

Medicare contractors are required to check CMS' master file of investigational devices that are eligible under this coverage. The file informs the contractor of the appropriate IDE number, related HCPCS codes (if applicable), and the start date, end date and maintenance date of the trial. The master file also includes a description of the device. Contractors must deny claims that do not include the IDE number assigned to the device, or where the date of service falls outside of the start and end dates for the trial.

As with the NCD, Medicare only pays for investigational devices when they are in certain clinical trials, in this case a clinical trial approved by the

FDA. The submission of a claim with the investigational device modifier is a certification by the provider that the FDA approved the clinical trial for the device.

 Are follow-up evaluative visits approved for payment after a Category B device is implanted?

 If the service pertains to an implant that falls under Category B IDE coverage, then follow-up visits would be covered. The coverage benefit includes care provided before, during, and after the procedure, so if the aftercare is related to the implant and is part of the protocol, then it would be covered and treated just like any other claim processed under this coverage. Also submit a copy of the approval letter substantiating the claim to payment if a different site submits the claim.

 Do the regulations differ when you are performing outpatient billing?

 Yes, they do. In 2002, CMS developed three G codes for use in reporting services furnished in hospital outpatient departments under national clinical trials. CMS created the codes because it felt it needed a more accurate method to separate the experimental intervention, which is not covered, from the routine cost items and services required solely because of the intervention, which are covered. These codes include the following:

- G0292—Administration(s) of experimental drug(s) only in a Medicare-qualifying clinical trial (includes administration for chemotherapy and other types of therapy via infusion and/or other than infusion), per day

- G0293—Noncovered surgical procedure(s) using conscious sedation, regional, general or spinal anesthesia in a Medicare qualifying clinical trial per day

- G0294—Noncovered surgical procedure(s) using either no anesthesia or local anesthesia only, in a Medicare-qualifying clinical trial per day

According to CMS, bill code G0292 when only experimental drugs are administered as part of a Medicare qualifying clinical trial. Don't use G0292 when an experimental drug is being administered in conjunction with payable drugs or on the same day as payable drugs. Instead, the appropriate drug administration code should be billed.

Similarly because procedures performed in the hospital outpatient department as part of a qualifying clinical trial are not covered under Medicare's clinical trial policy, CMS developed two G codes G0293 and G0294 to pay the hospital for its covered fixed costs associated with providing the service under the clinical trial.

If your hospital wants codes G0292, G0293 and G0294 to appear on a bill, ICD-9 diagnosis code V70.7 must be reported on the claim as a diagnosis other than the primary diagnosis. All three of these codes are for OPPS use only. Other provider types may not bill these codes.

The health care professional providing services would bill for his or her services on a HCFA-1500 and follow the modifier instructions discussed above.

 Does a LMRP supersede the clinical trial regulations or vice versa? For example, in a Phase III trial designed to compare the effectiveness of two FDA-approved drugs, there is already a LMRP saying Medicare will pay for the drug under study when administered for certain diagnoses. Since the NCD does not cover the study item or service, does this mean that Medicare will now not pay for the drug?

 The government has been very explicit regarding the NCD in terms of routine costs and its interactions with LMRPs. It says the NCD does not withdraw coverage for items and services that are covered under the LMRP.

 How should you bill Medicare when a patient in a clinical trial is randomized into the standard therapy control group in a device trial?

 Generally, the set of issues is the same whether the subject is in the experimental or control group. The same benefit category applies, as long as there are no statutory exclusions or national noncoverage decisions regarding these services, and as long as the services are reasonable and necessary. If those conditions are all same, it doesn't matter whether the subjects are in the control group.

 What modifiers should be used when billing for device benefits?

 See the answer to question #3.

We are a government agency hospital and receive flat-rate reimbursement on our inpatient cases. Our outpatient cases are subject to APCs or an itemized chart system. Have you seen rules implemented that create carve outs for noncovered services? How is that done in institutions like ours?

Medicare can make special "carve out" payments for high-cost items or services. That is typically negotiated with the government. This will require a fact-specific exchange with the program to determine what services are eligible for payment and how much payment they will receive. When you receive a protocol, it's important to start thinking about the billing and coding implications. Get a team assembled and write a memo that focuses on what items will be covered by the sponsor and which will be billed to Medicare. That memo should be given to the fiscal agent to ensure that he or she agrees with the approach you are taking. It's better to deal with these issues up front rather than on a crisis management basis.

What are the best practices for dealing with commercial payers?

When working with private payers, you need to plan and communicate with them before you start work, because often payment policies regarding coverage for clinical trials are very unclear and quite restrictive.

Begin by looking at your contract with the private payer. Make note of any exclusions. Often private payers will include clauses in the contract, but won't provide any of the related policies and procedures, so you are often bound by restrictions you haven't seen.

To secure reimbursement, start by writing to the major payers in your community and requesting copies of coverage policies with respect to trial-related services. If they are reluctant to provide those policies in writing, you may be able to set up a meeting to discuss any issues. Be certain to confirm any discussions in a certified letter mailed to the payer after that meeting.

I understand that the government will not pay any charges that are normally covered by sponsors, but I'm not sure how

to apply this in practical terms. Do you have any guidelines?

 The government inserted this provision to prevent sponsors from declining payment for services they have historically covered because Medicare is now willing to pick up the tab. This is a difficult area to navigate because it requires you to determine what items are typically covered by sponsors, not just at your facility, but throughout the clinical trials industry. Sponsors may negotiate different payments with different sites for the same or similar trials. You can take several steps to help address this requirement. Ask the sponsor about this issue. Also use your contacts at other research sites to address this. Asking for an assessment directly from the Medicare carrier or intermediary can also be helpful. As always, document the guidance you received in a letter back to the carrier or intermediary.

We primarily participate in research sponsored by pharmaceutical companies. How do we submit a protocol to CMS for approval?

Under the NCD you are not required to submit the protocol to the government. That said, however, the government could request to review the protocol if questions arose as to the propriety of the claims submitted to Medicare.

Appendix A

The Device Regulation—
42 CFR *Parts 405 and 411*

Appendix A

The Device Regulation—
42 CFR Parts 405 and 411

DEPARTMENT OF HEALTH AND HUMAN SERVICES
Health Care Financing Administration

42 *CFR* Parts 405 and 411

[BPD–841–FC]

RIN 0938–AH21

Medicare Program; Criteria and Procedures for Extending Coverage to
Certain Devices and Related Services

AGENCY: Health Care Financing Administration (HCFA), HHS.
ACTION: Final rule with comment period.

SUMMARY: This final rule establishes in regulations that certain devices
with an investigational device exemption (IDE) approved by the Food and
Drug Administration (FDA) and certain services related to those devices
may be covered under Medicare. Specifically, it sets forth the process by
which the FDA will assist HCFA in identifying non-experimental investigational devices that are potentially covered under Medicare.

Appendix A

This rule responds to the mandate that Federal agencies streamline their regulatory processes to make them less burdensome and more customer-focused. It is intended to provide Medicare beneficiaries with greater access to advances in medical technology and encourage clinical researchers to conduct high quality studies of newer technologies.

DATES: Effective Date: This rule is effective November 1, 1995.

Comment Date: Comments will be considered if we receive them at the appropriate address, as provided below, no later than 5 p.m. on November 20, 1995.

ADDRESSES: Mail written comments (1 original and 3 copies) to the following address:

Health Care Financing Administration, Department of Health and Human Services, Attention: BPD±841±FC, P.O. Box 26688, Baltimore, MD 21207±0519.

If you prefer, you may deliver your written comments (1 original and 3 copies) to one of the following addresses:

Room 309±G, Hubert H. Humphrey Building, 200 Independence Avenue, SW., Washington, DC 20201, or

Room C5±09±26, 7500 Security Boulevard, Baltimore, MD 21244± 1850.

Because of staffing and resource limitations, we cannot accept comments by facsimile (FAX) transmission. In commenting, please refer to file code BPD±841±FC. Comments received timely will be available for public inspection as they are received, generally beginning approximately 3 weeks after publication of a document, in Room 309±G of the Department's offices at 200 Independence Avenue, SW., Washington, DC, on Monday through Friday of each week from 8:30 a.m. to 5 p.m. (phone: (202) 690±7890).

Copies: To order copies of the Federal Register containing this document, send your request to: New Orders, Superintendent of Documents, P.O. Box 371954, Pittsburgh, PA 15250±7954. Specify the date of the issue requested and enclose a check or money order payable to the Superintendent of Documents, or enclose your Visa or Master Card number and expiration date. Credit card orders can also be placed by calling the order desk at (202) 512±1800 or by faxing to (202) 512± 2250. The cost for each copy is $8. As an alternative, you can view and photocopy the Federal Register document at most libraries designated as Federal Depository Libraries and at many other public and academic libraries throughout the country that receive the Federal Register .

FOR FURTHER INFORMATION CONTACT: Sharon Hippler, (410) 786±4633.

SUPPLEMENTARY INFORMATION:

I. Background

A. Statutory Basis

The Social Security Act (the Act) provides Medicare coverage for broad categories of benefits through the hospital insurance program, known as Part A, and the supplementary medical insurance program, known as Part B.

The Act does not, however, provide an all-inclusive list of covered items, services, treatments, procedures, or technologies. Except for certain items of durable medical equipment identified in section 1861(n) of the Act, some of the medical and other health services listed in section 1861(s) of the Act, and exclusions from coverage listed in section 1862 of the Act, the statute does not specify devices that are covered or excluded from coverage.

The Congress understood that questions about the coverage of specific services would invariably arise and would require a specific decision of coverage by the Secretary. Thus, it vested in the Secretary the authority to make those decisions. Among the provisions relevant to the determination of coverage is section 1862(a)(1)(A) of the Act, which states ``Notwithstanding any other provision of this title, no payment may be made under Part A or Part B for any expenses incurred for items or services which * * * are not reasonable and necessary for the diagnosis or treatment of illness or injury or to improve the functioning of a malformed body member.'' This is a key provision since the words ``notwithstanding any other provision of this title * * *'' make this an overriding exclusion that may be applicable in a given situation despite the existence of provisions that would otherwise permit coverage. Thus, while the Congress provided for the coverage of certain services, with limited exceptions specified by HCFA, coverage for those services is prohibited unless they are ``reasonable'' and ``necessary.''

B. Implementation of the Law

Historically, HCFA has interpreted the statutory terms ``reasonable'' and ``necessary'' to mean that a device must be safe and effective, medically necessary, and not experimental. For most Medicare coverage purposes, the term experimental has been used synonymously with the term investigational. Therefore, a device categorized by the FDA as being investigational served as an indication that it was not ``reasonable'' and ``necessary'' within the meaning of the Medicare program. As a general rule, these devices currently are not covered.

There is increasing recognition, however, that there are devices that are refinements of existing technologies or replications of existing technologies by other manufacturers. The FDA places many of these devices within the investigational device exemption (IDE) category as a means of gathering the scientific information necessary to establish the safety and effectiveness of the particular device, even though there is scientific evidence that similar devices can be safe and effective. Arguably, these devices could be viewed as ``reasonable'' and ``necessary'' under Medicare and recognized for payment if it were possible to identify them in the FDA's process.

C. January 1989 Proposed Rule on Coverage Decision Process

On January 30, 1989, we published a proposed rule (54 FR 4302) that proposed to establish in regulations generally applicable criteria for determining whether a service is ``reasonable'' and ``necessary'' under the Medicare program, and the coverage decisionmaking process. In response to that rule, we received comments pertaining to the coverage of experimental procedures and services related to those procedures. In this rule, we are choosing to respond to comments on investigational devices and services related to those devices and to announce our final policy. We have not completed our deliberations on the other issues addressed in the January 1989 proposed rule. This rule does not respond to comments other than those pertaining to devices.

Comment: Twenty-two commenters suggested that we revise our proposed policy so that we do not automatically exclude from Medicare coverage all devices that the FDA considers investigational. Several of these commenters recommended that we allow coverage of investigational devices when they are used in FDA-approved clinical trials.

Response: We agree that there are some investigational devices that should be considered for coverage if they are used in accordance with an FDA-approved protocol. The devices that will be considered for possible coverage are those investigational devices for which the FDA has determined that the device type can be safe and effective. For example, we will consider for possible coverage those investigational devices that are of the same type as a device for which a manufacturer has received FDA clearance or approval for marketing. We have entered into an interagency agreement with the FDA to identify those investigational devices that are of a device type for which the underlying questions of safety and effectiveness have been resolved. These devices may be covered if all other applicable Medicare coverage requirements are met.

Comment: One commenter recommended that we not change our previous policy that excluded coverage of investigational devices.

Response: We do not agree. We believe that there are certain investigational devices that should be covered if all other applicable coverage requirements are met. However, the investigational devices that we will consider for coverage will not include any device for which the FDA is unsure whether the device type in general can be safe and effective.

Comment: A number of commenters requested that we clarify the coverage rules concerning the furnishing of services related to experimental procedures (for example, a hospital stay).

Response: As stated earlier, we are limiting the focus of this rule to Medicare coverage of certain investigational devices and services related to those devices. Also, in the preamble to this rule and in new § 405.207, we explain our coverage policy concerning services related to a noncovered device.

II. Provisions of This Final Rule

While the policies contained in this final rule will be effective November 1, 1995, we are providing a 60-day comment period for the receipt of public comments. We believe it is appropriate to provide an opportunity for comment on these policies because we are broadening the proposals concerning certain devices contained in the January 1989 proposed rule. Consequently, beneficiaries, providers, and suppliers that may have chosen not to comment because they may have believed they were not affected by the 1989 proposals may wish to comment on these broadened final policies. If our consideration of the comments we receive leads us to a change in these policies, we will publish another document.

A. HCFA Coverage Decision Process

The Administration has set forth a mandate that all Federal agencies must streamline their regulatory processes to make them less burdensome and more customer-focused. Agencies have been directed to review their policies and processes to determine which requirements can be reduced or eliminated without lowering health and safety standards. In accordance with this directive, the FDA reviewed its regulatory processes for devices and HCFA reviewed its Medicare coverage policies. This rule results in an improved process for covering certain investigational devices that is expected to benefit Medicare beneficiaries.

This new policy will lead to broader coverage of certain investigational devices and certain services related to those devices. A long-term benefit is to facilitate the collection of information about these devices through approved clinical trials, which will enable the marketing of these devices. Medicare beneficiaries will have earlier access to the latest advances in medical technology.

To assist HCFA in its coverage decision process, the FDA will follow a categorization process that differentiates between the clinical assessment of novel, first-of-a-kind devices and newer generations of legally marketed devices. The policy changes in this rule reflect the categorization of investigational devices that are the subject of FDA-approved IDEs.

The FDA uses the definition of a device that appears in 21 U.S.C. 321(h). A device, for purposes of the FDA process, refers to an instrument, apparatus, implement, machine, contrivance, implant, in vitro reagent, or other similar or related article, including any component, part, or accessory, which is Ð

- Recognized in the official National Formulary, or the U.S. Pharmacopeia, or any supplement to them,
- Intended for use in the diagnosis of disease or other conditions, or in the cure, mitigation, treatment, or prevention of disease, in man or other animals,
- Intended for use in the diagnosis of conditions other than diseases such as pregnancy,
- Intended to affect the structure or any function of the body of man or other animals, or
- Considered an in vitro diagnostic product, including those previously regulated as drugs, and which does not achieve any of its principal intended purposes through chemical action within or on the body of man or other animals

and which is not dependent upon being metabolized for the achievement of any of its principal intended purposes.

When a sponsor (usually a manufacturer) submits a marketing application for clearance or approval of a device to the FDA, the FDA evaluates the safety and effectiveness of the device. If sufficient information exists to determine its safety and effectiveness, the FDA may clear the device for marketing. In some instances, for certain devices, the FDA may require that clinical trials be conducted to obtain clinical information to determine the device's safety and effectiveness. Generally, in order for these devices to be shipped lawfully for purposes of conducting the clinical trial, the sponsor must obtain an approved investigational device exemption (IDE).

Under the Food, Drug, and Cosmetic Act (21 U.S.C. 360c), devices fall into one of three classes:

Class IÐDevices for which the general controls of the Food, Drug, and Cosmetic Act, such as adherence to good manufacturing practice regulations, are sufficient to provide a reasonable assurance of safety and effectiveness.

Class IIÐDevices that, in addition to general controls, require special controls, such as performance standards or postmarket surveillance, to provide a reasonable assurance of safety and effectiveness.

Class IIIÐDevices that cannot be classified into Class I or Class II because insufficient information exists to determine that either special or general controls would provide reasonable assurance of safety and effectiveness. Class III devices require premarket approval.

Under the new categorization process to assist HCFA, the FDA assigns each device with an FDA-approved IDE to one of two categories: Experimental/ Investigational (Category A) Devices, or Non-Experimental/Investigational (Category B) Devices. Under this categorization process, an experimental/ investigational device (Category A) is an innovative device in Class III for which ``absolute risk'' of the device type has not been established (that is, initial questions of safety and effectiveness have not been resolved and the FDA is unsure whether the device type can be safe and effective). A non-experimental/ investigational (Category B) device is a device believed to be in Class I or Class II, or a device believed to be in Class III for which the incremental risk is the primary risk in question (that is, underlying questions of safety and effectiveness of that device type have been resolved), or it is known that the device type can be safe and effective because, for example, other manufacturers have obtained FDA approval for that device type. The criteria the FDA will use to categorize an investigational device is described in the addendum to this rule.

Currently there are about 1,200 FDA-approved clinical trials of devices. The FDA is categorizing those devices as ``experimental/investigational (Category A)'' or ``non-experimental/investigational (Category B),'' a process that is expected to be completed by November 1, 1995. The great majority of these devices in clinical trials are likely to be categorized as ``non-experimental/investigational (Category B)''.

The FDA will notify HCFA, when it notifies the sponsor, either by electronic means or written communication, of its categorization decisions. Through these categorization decisions, the FDA will be advising HCFA as to the similarity of a device that has been approved for use in an FDA-approved clinical trial to a device that has been approved or cleared by the FDA for marketing.

HCFA excludes from Medicare coverage a device with an IDE that is categorized by the FDA as experimental/investigational (Category A). HCFA will continue to view these experimental/investigational (Category A) devices as not satisfying the statutory requirement that Medicare pay for only devices determined to be reasonable and necessary. HCFA is not changing its policy on this issue because essential considerations of health and safety are involved.

This rule does not affect HCFA's policy on services related to a noncovered device. That is, services related to the use of a noncovered device are not covered under Medicare. We are codifying in the regulations a provision explaining that services related to a noncovered device are not covered under Medicare. These services include all services furnished in preparation for the use of a noncovered device, services furnished contemporaneously with and necessary to the use of a noncovered device, and services furnished as necessary after-care that are incident to recovery from the use of the device or from receiving related noncovered services.

Services furnished to address medical complications arising from the use of the device (and that are not incident to normal recovery) may be covered. Services not related to the use of a noncovered device, which meet all other coverage requirements, can be covered under Medicare.

The following are some examples of services ``related to'' and ``not related to'' noncovered devices furnished while the beneficiary is an inpatient:

• A beneficiary is hospitalized to receive a noncovered device and breaks a leg while in the hospital. Services

related to care of the broken leg during this stay are ``not related to'' services and are covered under Medicare.

• A beneficiary is admitted to the hospital for a covered service and during the hospital stay received a noncovered investigational device. The services related to the admitting condition are covered because the reason for the admission was to receive covered services and not related to the diagnoses that led to the need for the noncovered device.

• A beneficiary is admitted to the hospital for covered services related to a condition that led to receiving a noncovered device during the same hospital stay. We would review all of the services and make a comparison of the date they are received to the date the beneficiary is identified as needing the noncovered device. If our review reveals that services were required because of receiving the noncovered device, the services ``related to'' the noncovered device will not be covered.

• After a beneficiary is discharged from a hospital stay during which he or she receives a noncovered investigational device, medical and hospital services to treat a condition or complication that arises as a result of the noncovered device or related noncovered services may be covered when they are reasonable and necessary in all other respects. Thus, coverage could be provided for subsequent inpatient hospital stays or outpatient treatment ordinarily covered by Medicare, even if the need for treatment arose because of a previous noncovered device or related noncovered services. Any subsequent services that could be expected to have been incorporated into a global fee, however, will not be covered.

The related services policy will also apply to experimental/investigational (Category A) and non-experimental/investigational (Category B) devices that are excluded from Medicare coverage. Therefore, Medicare policy will continue to preclude coverage of certain devices and services related to the use of those devices when they are furnished as part of a hospital stay.

It is our intention that a beneficiary not pay for a noncovered device or services related to a noncovered device when a beneficiary did not know that the device or related services are not covered. Existing regulations concerning limitations on liability in §§ 411.400 through 411.406 will apply to this broader coverage of certain investigational devices and services related to those devices. Medicare payment may be made for certain assigned claims for a service related to

a noncovered device if the service was excluded from coverage in accordance with § 411.15(k) as not medically necessary under section 1862(a)(1)(A) of the Act. A beneficiary who did not know and could not reasonably have been expected to know that payment would be denied under section 1862(a)(1)(A) of the Act receives protection from financial liability in accordance with §§ 411.400 through 411.406 under the limitation on liability provision of section 1879 of the Act. Similarly, when the beneficiary is protected and the provider or supplier also did not know and could not reasonably have been expected to know that payment would be denied, the provider or supplier also receives protection from financial liability in accordance with the limitation on liability provision. Consequently, Medicare payment may be made to the provider or supplier.

For unassigned claims for related physician services excluded from coverage as not medically necessary under section 1862(a)(1)(A) of the Act, a beneficiary who did not know and could not reasonably have been expected to know that payment would be denied as not medically necessary may receive protection from financial liability in accordance with existing § 411.408 under the refund requirement provision of section 1842(l) of the Act. If the beneficiary is found not to have known, and the provider or supplier also did not know and could not reasonably have been expected to know that payment would be denied, the provider or supplier will receive protection from financial liability under the refund requirement provision.

Under changes made by this final rule, HCFA will consider coverage of a device with an FDA-approved IDE, categorized by the FDA as non-experimental/investigational (Category B) for Medicare beneficiaries participating in FDA-approved clinical trials. As a general rule for all medical care, HCFA has authority to conduct a separate assessment of an itemÐs or service's appropriateness for Medicare coverage, including whether it is reasonable and necessary specifically for its intended use for Medicare beneficiaries. Medicare coverage of a non-experimental/investigational (Category B) device will be subject to the same process and criteria used by Medicare contractors when making coverage decisions for legally marketed devices. Coverage of the device is dependent on it meeting all other Medicare coverage requirements contained in the statute, regulations, and instructions issued by HCFA.

The FDA-approved IDE study protocols restrict investigational device shipment to a limited number of investigational sites for testing on a specific number of patients. To the extent Medicare covers a non-experimental/investigational (Category B) device, coverage is limited to beneficiaries meeting the protocol requirements. For example, coverage of an investigational device may be limited to Medicare beneficiaries participating in trials conducted by certain health care practitioners in an approved clinical trial.

Medicare coverage of a non-experimental/investigational (Category B) device is predicated, in part, upon the device continuing to meet criteria that led to this designation by the FDA. In the event a device fails to meet the criteria for Category B designation or its use violates relevant IDE requirements necessitating the withdrawal of the IDE approval, the FDA will immediately notify the sponsor and HCFA. HCFA will re-evaluate the device's continued eligibility for Medicare payment.

Payment under Medicare for a non-experimental/investigational (Category B) device will be based on, and may not exceed, the amount that would have been paid for a currently used device serving the same medical purpose that has been approved or cleared for marketing by the FDA. In cases involving a hospital stay, the diagnosis related group (DRG) payment under the prospective payment system ordinarily will not be affected.

B. Re-evaluation of Categorization Decision

We anticipate that instances will arise under which a device sponsor believes that a device, categorized by the FDA as experimental/investigational (Category A), should be categorized as non-experimental/investigational (Category B). In these instances, the sponsor may request that the FDA re-evaluate its categorization decision. Only after the FDA has completed its re-evaluation, and concluded that the device still is an experimental/investigational (Category A) device, may a sponsor request review by HCFA. A sponsor may request review by HCFA even if no Medicare claims are involved.

1. FDA Action

Under this process, the sponsor may submit a written request for re-evaluation to the FDA (at the same address it submitted its original application), together with information and rationale that it believes support recategorization. Only the sponsor of a device may seek a re-evaluation of the FDA IDE categorization decision.

Time limits on seeking a re-evaluation will not be imposed. The FDA will review the request and inform the sponsor, and HCFA, of its decision. If the FDA does not agree to recategorize the device, the sponsor may seek further review by HCFA.

2. HCFA Action

Upon written request to the HCFA Administrator from the sponsor of a device with an FDA-approved IDE, HCFA will review the categorization of the device. As part of this process, HCFA will review all information submitted by the sponsor and the FDA's recommendation. HCFA will review only information in the FDA record to determine whether to change the categorization. HCFA will not accept or review any information from the sponsor that was not previously reviewed by the FDA. While HCFA, during the re-evaluation process, will be the final decisionmaker concerning categorization of a device for Medicare coverage purposes, HCFA relies heavily on the FDA review of the scientific information related to the device and consequently the FDA recommendation. HCFA will issue a written decision and notify the sponsor and the FDA. No further reviews will be available to the sponsor.

3. Update of Categorization Decision

If the circumstances that led to the initial categorization decision change (for example, a premarket approval application is approved for a device similar to one under investigation), the FDA will re-evaluate the categorization designation and notify the sponsor and HCFA of any change. Neither the FDA categorization and re-evaluation nor HCFA's review constitute an initial determination for purposes of the Medicare appeals processes under 42 CFR part 405, subparts G or H, or parts 417, 473, or 498.

C. Quarterly Announcement of Categorization Decisions

HCFA publishes quarterly in the Federal Register a notice that lists HCFA manual instructions, substantive and interpretive regulations and other Federal Register notices, and statements of policy that relate to the Medicare and Medicaid programs. HCFA will announce in the quarterly notice all IDE categorizations, using IDE numbers the FDA assigns. The initial notice will include all FDA-approved IDE numbers organized by the categories to which the device numbers are assigned (that is, Category A or Category B, and identified by the IDE number). Subsequent notices will include the additions and deletions to the initial list of all devices with an FDA-approved IDE.

D. Confidentiality of Investigational Device Exemption Information

Data and information otherwise exempt from public disclosure may be revealed in judicial proceedings if the data or information are relevant. HCFA will take appropriate measures, or request that appropriate measures be taken, to reduce disclosure to the minimum necessary under the circumstances. Because HCFA relies on information submitted to the FDA under 21 U.S.C. 360j(g), HCFA will consult with the FDA to ensure that the confidentiality of the information is protected to the extent possible.

E. Contractor Coverage Decisions of Devices With an FDA-approved IDE

1. Current Contractor Functions

Sections 1816 and 1842 of the Act provide for most claims processing and administrative functions for Medicare to be handled by public or private insurance organizations (commercial insurers or Blue Cross/Blue Shield Associations) acting as fiscal agents or contractors for the Medicare program. The contractors responsible for the administration of Part A benefits are called fiscal intermediaries. The major role of the intermediaries is to review and pay claims submitted by providers (such as hospitals, skilled nursing facilities, and home health agencies) for covered services furnished to Medicare beneficiaries. The intermediary makes payments for hospital inpatient services generally under the prospective payment system. It makes payments for hospital and other provider outpatient services by reviewing submitted cost reports and making reasonable cost determinations or payment determinations under a fee schedule following policies set by HCFA.

Under Part B, the contractors are called carriers. Part B services are paid on a fee schedule, reasonable charge, or reasonable cost basis. One of the major functions of the carriers is to determine the appropriate amount of payment for each medical care service paid for under the program. Carriers also are responsible for reviewing and paying claims to or on behalf of beneficiaries for the services furnished.

The functions performed by Medicare contractors include utilization review, beneficiary hearings and appeals, professional relations, and statistical activities, in addition to claims review and processing. Currently, there are 29

Appendix A

carriers, 46 intermediaries, and some other entities under contract with HCFA that perform reviews and process claims for Medicare beneficiaries.

2. Current Criteria and Procedures for Contractor Coverage Decisions

Contractors make Medicare coverage decisions within the parameters set by statutory authority and regulations and program instructions issued by HCFA. If HCFA has issued a national coverage decision, contractors are bound by that decision. If no national coverage decision has been issued, a contractor must decide whether the service in question is reasonable and necessary and therefore covered by Medicare.

Medicare contractors may specifically consider, among other factors, whether the service isÐ

• Medically necessary in the particular case and whether the amount, duration, and frequency of use or application of the service are medically appropriate;

• Furnished in accordance with accepted standards of medical practice; and

• Furnished in a setting appropriate to the patient's medical needs and condition (such as inpatient care at a hospital or skilled nursing facility, outpatient care at a hospital or physician's office, or home care).

3. Changes to Contractor Process

Under this rule, contractors will review the instructions HCFA issues to determine if a non-experimental/investigational (Category B) device is potentially covered under Medicare. After determining that a device is potentially covered, the contractor will apply HCFA's long-standing criteria and procedures for making coverage decisions. When considering whether a non-experimental/investigational (Category B) device is furnished in accordance with accepted standards of medical practice, it will consider those standards that relate to an FDA-approved clinical trial.

In accordance with HCFA coverage policy, Medicare contractors are precluded from covering any device that is an experimental/investigational (Category A) device.

F. Appeals Under Part A and Part B

While the categorization decision is not itself an initial determination, if HCFA denies a Medicare claim on the basis that the device is an experimental/investigational (Category A) device, the initial determination denying the claim encompasses the categorization decision. A proper party to the denied Medicare claim has a right to appeal the experimental/investigational (Category A) categorization as an initial determination under 42 CFR part 405, subparts G or H.

A decision that a device is experimental/investigational (Category A) means that the device is experimental and, therefore, excluded from coverage as not reasonable and necessary under section 1862(a)(1)(A) of the Act. HCFA's acceptance of the FDA categorization of an experimental/investigational (Category A) device constitutes a national coverage decision and is binding on HCFA's contractors. In accordance with section 1869(b)(3)(A) of the Act, national coverage decisions made by HCFA under section 1862(a)(1) of the Act may not be reviewed by administrative law judges.

III. Regulatory Impact Statement

Consistent with the Regulatory Flexibility Act (RFA) (5 U.S.C. 601 through 612), we prepare a regulatory flexibility analysis unless we certify that a rule will not have a significant economic impact on a substantial number of small entities. For purposes of the RFA, all device manufacturers and providers are considered to be small entities. Individuals and States are not included in the definition of a small entity.

In addition, section 1102(b) of the Act requires us to prepare a regulatory impact analysis if a rule may have a significant impact on the operations of a substantial number of small rural hospitals. This analysis must conform to the provisions of section 604 of the RFA. For purposes of section 1102(b) of the Act, we define a small rural hospital as a hospital that is located outside of a Metropolitan Statistical Area and has fewer than 50 beds.

This regulation removes certain investigational devices from being presumed excluded by Medicare and places them in a category under which they may be covered. On a claim-by-claim basis, Medicare contractors verify or determine that devices are covered under the circumstances presented by the claim or bill. This regulation does not change that process, except the contractors must ascertain whether these devices were furnished to beneficiaries participating in, and in accordance with the requirements of, approved clinical trials. Once coverage is verified, payment is made at the level established for a similar device that has been approved as covered by Medicare.

We anticipate that this regulation will lead to a beneficial but not a major expansion of coverage of devices. Each year the FDA receives approximately 200 IDE applications for review. The majority of these IDEs are approved for study. At the present time, there are approximately 1,200 clinical trials underway involving devices, which are being conducted under FDA-approved IDEs.

We expect that this regulation will have a number of beneficial effects. It will provide Medicare beneficiaries with greater access to advances in medical technology. It will allow Medicare beneficiaries faced with a decision of choosing between a fully covered device and one undergoing clinical trials to choose the investigational device without losing Medicare coverage. Because Medicare payment is based on the payment for a fully covered device, that choice would not result in increased costs to Medicare for those devices.

At the present time, device manufacturers and the providers that furnish services involving non-experimental/investigational devices (Category B) are not eligible for Medicare payments. We estimate that this regulation will result in negligible costs to the Medicare program. We expect affected entities would receive less than $10 million per year over the next 5 years.

Virtually all of these devices replace devices for which Medicare coverage is currently available and which would have been furnished to beneficiaries if we had not changed the policy. The services are primarily furnished on an inpatient basis in hospitals. Hospitals are paid on a prospective basis so that prices are not adjusted based on changes in the price-components (that is, device costs) of individual DRGs. Instead, the payment base under the prospective payment system is annually updated based on a host of considerations, including the increased cost of inputs. As a result, this change in coverage will not significantly affect Medicare's current payments and will only affect its future payments in concert with the other factors affecting the DRG update decisions.

For these reasons, we are not preparing analyses for either the RFA or section 1102(b) of the Act because we have determined, and we certify, that this rule will not have a significant economic impact on a substantial number of small entities or a significant impact on the operations of a substantial number of small rural hospitals.

In accordance with the provisions of Executive Order 12866, this regulation was reviewed by the Office of Management and Budget.

IV. Collection of Information Requirements

This document does not impose information collection and recordkeeping requirements. Consequently, it need not be reviewed by the Office of Management and Budget under the authority of the Paperwork Reduction Act of 1980 (44 U.S.C. 3501 et seq.).

V. Response to Comments

Because of the large number of items of correspondence we normally receive on Federal Register documents published for comment, we are not able to acknowledge or respond to them individually. We will consider all comments we receive by the date and time specified in the ``DATES'' section of this preamble, and, if we proceed with a subsequent document, we will respond to the comments in the preamble to that document.

List of Subjects

42 CFR Part 405

Administrative practice and procedure, Health facilities, Health professions, Kidney diseases, Medicare, Reporting and recordkeeping requirements, Rural areas, X-rays.

42 CFR Part 411

Kidney diseases, Medicare, Reporting and recordkeeping requirements.

For the reasons set forth in the preamble, 42 CFR Chapter IV is amended as follows:
A. 42 CFR part 405 is amended to read as follows:

PART 405—FEDERAL HEALTH INSURANCE FOR THE AGED AND DISABLED

1. A new subpart B, consisting of §§ 405.201±405.215, is added to read as follows:

Subpart B—Medical Services Coverage Decisions That Relate to Health Care Technology

Sec.
405.201   Scope of subpart and definitions.
405.203   FDA categorization of investigational devices.
405.205   Coverage of a non-experimental/ investigational (Category B) device.
405.207   Services related to a noncovered device.
405.209   Payment for a non-experimental/ investigational (Category B) device.
405.211   Procedures for Medicare contractors in making coverage decisions for a non-experimental/investigational (Category B) device.
405.213   Re-evaluation of a device categorization.
405.215   Confidential commercial and trade secret information.

Subpart B—Medical Services Coverage Decisions That Relate to Health Care Technology

Authority: Secs. 1102, 1862, and 1871 of the Social Security Act as amended (42 U.S.C. 1302, 1395y, and 1395hh).

§ 405.201   Scope of subpart and definitions.

(a) Scope. This subpart establishes thatÐ
(1) HCFA uses the FDA categorization of a device as a factor in making Medicare coverage decisions; and
(2) HCFA may consider for Medicare coverage certain devices with an FDA-approved investigational device exemption (IDE) that have been categorized as non-experimental/ investigational (Category B).
(b) Definitions. As used in this subpartÐ
Class I refers to devices for which the general controls of the Food, Drug, and Cosmetic Act, such as adherence to good manufacturing practice regulations, are sufficient to provide a reasonable assurance of safety and effectiveness.
Class II refers to devices that, in addition to general controls, require special controls, such as performance standards or postmarket surveillance, to provide a reasonable assurance of safety and effectiveness.
Class III refers to devices that cannot be classified into Class I or Class II because insufficient information exists to determine that either special or general controls would provide reasonable assurance of safety and effectiveness. Class III devices require premarket approval.
Contractors refers to carriers, fiscal intermediaries, and other entities that contract with HCFA to review and adjudicate claims for Medicare services.
Experimental/investigational (Category A) device refers to an innovative device believed to be in Class III for which ``absolute risk'' of the device type has not been established (that is, initial questions of safety and effectiveness have not been resolved and the FDA is unsure whether the device type can be safe and effective).
IDE stands for investigational device exemption. An FDA-approved IDE application permits a device, which would otherwise be subject to marketing clearance, to be shipped lawfully for the purpose of conducting a clinical trial in accordance with 21 U.S.C. 360j(g) and 21 CFR parts 812 and 813.
Non-experimental/investigational (Category B) device refers to a device believed to be in Class I or Class II, or a device believed to be in Class III for

which the incremental risk is the primary risk in question (that is, underlying questions of safety and effectiveness of that device type have been resolved), or it is known that the device type can be safe and effective because, for example, other manufacturers have obtained FDA approval for that device type.
PMA stands for ``premarket approval'' and refers to a marketing application for a Class III device, which includes all information submitted with or incorporated by reference in the application in accordance with 21 U.S.C. 360e and 360j and 21 CFR 814.3(e).
Sponsor refers to a person or entity that initiates, but does not conduct, an investigation under an IDE.

§ 405.203   FDA categorization of investigational devices.

(a) The FDA assigns a device with an FDA-approved IDE to one of two categories:
(1) Experimental/Investigational (Category A) Devices.
(2) Non-Experimental/Investigational (Category B) Devices.
(b) The FDA notifies HCFA, when it notifies the sponsor, that the device is categorized by FDA as experimental/ investigational (Category A) or non-experimental/investigational (Category B).
(c) HCFA uses the categorization of the device as a factor in making Medicare coverage decisions.

§ 405.205   Coverage of a non-experimental/ investigational (Category B) device.

(a) For any device that meets the requirements of the exception at § 411.15(o) of this chapter, the following procedures apply:
(1) The FDA notifies HCFA, when it notifies the sponsor, that the device is categorized by FDA as non-experimental/investigational (Category B).
(2) HCFA uses the categorization of the device as a factor in making Medicare coverage decisions.
(b) If the FDA becomes aware that a categorized device no longer meets the requirements of the exception at § 411.15(o) of this chapter, the FDA notifies the sponsor and HCFA and the procedures described in paragraph (a)(2) of this section apply.

§ 405.207   Services related to a noncovered device.

(a) When payment is not made. Medicare payment is not made for medical and hospital services that are related to the use of a device that is not covered because HCFA determines the device is not ``reasonable'' and

Appendix A

``necessary'' under section 1862(a)(1)(A) of the Act or because it is excluded from coverage for other reasons. These services include all services furnished in preparation for the use of a noncovered device, services furnished contemporaneously with and necessary to the use of a noncovered device, and services furnished as necessary after-care that are incident to recovery from the use of the device or from receiving related noncovered services.

(b) When payment is made. Medicare payment may be made for services, ordinarily covered by Medicare, to treat a condition or complication that arises because of the use of a noncovered device or from the furnishing of related noncovered services.

§ 405.209   Payment for a non-experimental/investigational (Category B) device.

Payment under Medicare for a non-experimental/investigational (Category B) device is based on, and may not exceed, the amount that would have been paid for a currently used device serving the same medical purpose that has been approved or cleared for marketing by the FDA.

§ 405.211   Procedures for Medicare contractors in making coverage decisions for a non-experimental/investigational (Category B) device.

(a) General rule. In their review of claims for payment, Medicare contractors are bound by the statute, regulations, and all HCFA administrative issuances, including all national coverage decisions.

(b) Potentially covered non-experimental/investigational (Category B) devices. Medicare contractors may approve coverage for any device with an FDA-approved IDE categorized as a non-experimental/investigational (Category B) device if all other coverage requirements are met.

(c) Other considerations. Medicare contractors must consider whether any restrictions concerning site of service, indications for use, or any other list of conditions for coverage have been placed on the device's use.

§ 405.213   Re-evaluation of a device categorization.

(a) General rules. (1) Any sponsor that does not agree with an FDA decision that categorizes its device as experimental/investigational (Category A) may request re-evaluation of the categorization decision.

(2) A sponsor may request review by HCFA only after the requirements of paragraph (b) of this section are met.

(3) No reviews other than those described in paragraphs (b) and (c) of this section are available to the sponsor.

(4) Neither the FDA original categorization or re-evaluation (described in paragraph (b) of this section) nor HCFA's review (described in paragraph (c) of this section) constitute an initial determination for purposes of the Medicare appeals processes under part 405, subpart G or subpart H, or parts 417, 473, or 498 of this chapter.

(b) Request to FDA. A sponsor that does not agree with the FDA's categorization of its device may submit a written request to the FDA at any time requesting re-evaluation of its original categorization decision, together with any information and rationale that it believes support recategorization. The FDA notifies both HCFA and the sponsor of its decision.

(c) Request to HCFA. If the FDA does not agree to recategorize the device, the sponsor may seek review from HCFA. A device sponsor must submit its request in writing to HCFA. HCFA obtains copies of relevant portions of the application, the original categorization decision, and supplementary materials. HCFA reviews all material submitted by the sponsor and the FDA's recommendation. HCFA reviews only information in the FDA record to determine whether to change the categorization of the device. HCFA issues a written decision and notifies the sponsor of the IDE and the FDA.

§ 405.215   Confidential commercial and trade secret information.

To the extent that HCFA relies on confidential commercial or trade secret information in any judicial proceeding, HCFA will maintain confidentiality of the information in accordance with Federal law.

Subpart G—[Amended]

2. The authority citation for subpart G continues to read as follows:

Authority: Secs. 1102, 1151, 1154, 1155, 1869(b), 1871, 1872, and 1879 of the Social Security Act (42 U.S.C. 1302, 1320c, 1320c± 3, 1320c±4, 1395ff(b), 1395hh, 1395ii and 1395pp).

3. In subpart G, a new § 405.753 is added to read as follows:

§ 405.753   Appeal of a categorization of a device.

(a) HCFA's acceptance of the FDA categorization of a device as an experimental/investigational (Category A) device under § 405.203 is a national coverage decision under section 1862(a)(1) of the Act.

(b) HCFA's acceptance of the FDA categorization of a device as an experimental/investigational (Category A) device under § 405.203 is an aspect

of an initial determination that, under section 1862 of the Act, payment may not be made.

(c) In accordance with section 1869(b)(3)(A) of the Act, HCFA's acceptance of the FDA categorization of a device as an experimental/investigational (Category A) device under § 405.203 may not be reviewed by an administrative law judge.

Subpart H—[Amended]

4. The authority citation for subpart H continues to read as follows:

Authority: Secs. 1102, 1842(b)(3)(C), and 1869(b) of the Social Security Act (42 U.S.C. 1302, 1395u(b)(3)(C), 1395ff(b)).

5. In subpart H, a new § 405.877 is added to read as follows:

§ 405.877   Appeal of a categorization of a device.

(a) HCFA's acceptance of the FDA categorization of a device as an experimental/investigational (Category A) device under § 405.203 is a national coverage decision under section 1862(a)(1) of the Act.

(b) HCFA's acceptance of the FDA categorization of a device as an experimental/investigational (Category A) device under § 405.203 is an aspect of an initial determination that, under section 1862 of the Act, payment may not be made.

(c) In accordance with section 1869(b)(3)(A) of the Act, HCFA's acceptance of the FDA categorization of a device as an experimental/investigational (Category A) device under § 405.203 may not be reviewed by an administrative law judge.

B. 42 CFR part 411 is amended as set forth below:

PART 411—EXCLUSIONS FROM MEDICARE AND LIMITATIONS ON MEDICARE PAYMENT

1. The authority citation for part 411 continues to read as follows:

Authority: Secs. 1102 and 1871 of the Social Security Act (42 U.S.C. 1302 and 1395hh).

2. In § 411.15, the introductory text is republished and new paragraph (o) is added to read as follows:

§ 411.15   Particular services excluded from coverage.

The following services are excluded from coverage.

*   *   *   *   *

(o) Experimental or investigational devices, except for certain devicesÐ

(1) Categorized by the FDA as a non-experimental/investigational (Category B) device defined in § 405.201(b) of this chapter; and

(2) Furnished in accordance with the FDA-approved protocols governing clinical trials.

3. In § 411.406, paragraph (e) is revised to read as follows:

§ 411.406 Criteria for determining that a provider, practitioner, or supplier knew that services were excluded from coverage as custodial care or as not reasonable and necessary.

*   *   *   *   *

(e) Knowledge based on experience, actual notice, or constructive notice   . It is clear that the provider, practitioner, or supplier could have been expected to have known that the services were excluded from coverage on the basis of the following:

(1) Its receipt of HCFA notices, including manual issuances, bulletins, or other written guides or directives from intermediaries, carriers, or PROs, including notification of PRO screening criteria specific to the condition of the beneficiary for whom the furnished services are at issue and of medical procedures subject to preadmission review by a PRO.

(2) Federal Register publications containing notice of national coverage decisions or of other specifications regarding noncoverage of an item or service.

(3) Its knowledge of what are considered acceptable standards of practice by the local medical community.

(Catalog of Federal Domestic Assistance Program No. 93.773, MedicareÐHospital Insurance; and Program No. 93.774, MedicareÐSupplementary Medical Insurance Program)

Dated: September 11, 1995.

Bruce C. Vladeck,

Administrator, Health Care Financing Administration.

Dated: September 12, 1995.

Donna E. Shalala,

Secretary.

Note: This addendum will not appear in the Code of Federal Regulations.

AddendumÐCriteria for Categorization of Investigational Devices

Category A: Experimental/ Investigational

Category A devices include the following:

(1) Class III devices of a type for which no marketing application has been approved through the premarket approval (PMA) process for any indication for use. (For pre-amendments [1] Class III devices, refer to the criteria under Category B).

(2) Class III devices that would otherwise be in Category B but have undergone significant modification for a new indication for use.

Category B: Non-experimental/ Investigational

Category B devices include the following:

(1) Devices, regardless of the classification, under investigation to establish substantial equivalence to a predicate device, that is, to establish substantial equivalence to a previously/ currently legally marketed device.

(2) Class III devices whose technological characteristics and indications for use are comparable to a PMA-approved device.

(3) Class III devices with technological advances compared to a PMA-approved device, that is, a device with technological changes that represent advances to a device that has already received PMA-approval (generational changes).

(4) Class III devices that are comparable to a PMA-approved device but are under investigation for a new indication for use. For purposes of studying the new indication, no significant modifications to the device were required.

(5) Pre-amendments Class III devices that become the subject of an IDE after the FDA requires premarket approval, that is, no PMA application was submitted or the PMA application was denied.

(6) Nonsignificant risk device investigations for which the FDA required the submission of an IDE.

Note: Some investigational devices may exhibit unique characteristics or raise safety concerns that make additional consideration necessary. For these devices, HCFA and the FDA will agree on the additional criteria to be used. The FDA will use these criteria to assign the device(s) to a category. As experience is gained in the categorization process, this addendum may be modified.

[FR Doc. 95±23132 Filed 9±13±95; 4:00 pm]

BILLING CODE 4120–01–P

---

[1] Pre-amendments devices are devices that were marketed before the enactment of the 1976 Medical Device Amendments to the Food, Drug, and Cosmetic Act; that is, in commercial distribution before May 28, 1976.

Source: September 19, 1995 Federal Register, *Vol. 60, No. 181.*

Appendix B

The Final National Coverage Decision

Appendix B

Medicare Coverage: Clinical Trials

Final National Coverage Decision

This national coverage policy is based upon the authority found in §1862(a)(1)(E) of the Social Security Act (Act). It is binding on all Medicare carriers, fiscal intermediaries, Peer Review Organizations, Health Maintenance Organizations, Competitive Medical Plans, Health Care Prepayment Plans, and Medicare+Choice organizations (§1852(a)(1)(A) of the Act). In addition, an administrative law judge may not disregard, set aside, or otherwise review a national coverage decision issued under §1862(a)(1) of the Act. 42 C.F.R. §405.860.

Clinical Trials

Effective for items and services furnished on or after September 19, 2000, Medicare covers the routine costs of qualifying clinical trials, as such costs are defined below, as well as reasonable and necessary items and services used to diagnose and treat complications arising from participation in all clinical trials. All other Medicare rules apply.

Routine costs of a clinical trial include all items and services that are otherwise generally available to Medicare beneficiaries (i.e., there exists a benefit category, it is not statutorily excluded, and there is not a national noncoverage decision) that are provided in either the experimental or the control arms of a clinical trial except:

- the investigational item or service, itself,

- items and services provided solely to satisfy data collection and analysis needs and that are not used in the direct clinical management of the patient (e.g., monthly CT scans for a condition usually requiring only a single scan); and

- items and services customarily provided by the research sponsors free of charge for any enrollee in the trial.

Routine costs in clinical trials include:

- Items or services that are typically provided absent a clinical trial (e.g., conventional care);

- Items or services required solely for the provision of the investigational item or service (e.g., administration of a noncovered chemotherapeutic agent), the clinically appropriate monitoring of the effects of the item or service, or the prevention of complications; and

- Items or services needed for reasonable and necessary care arising from the provision of an investigational item or service--in particular, for the diagnosis or treatment of complications.

This policy does not withdraw Medicare coverage for items and services that may be covered according to local medical review policies or the regulations on Category B investigational device exemptions (IDE) found in 42 C.F.R. §405.201-405.215 and §411.15 and §411.406. For information about LMRPs, refer to www.lmrp.net, a searchable database of Medicare contractors' local policies.

For noncovered items and services, including items and services for which Medicare payment is statutorily prohibited, Medicare only covers the treat- ment of complications arising from the delivery of the noncovered item or service and unrelated reasonable and necessary care. (Refer to MCM 2300.1 and MIM 3101.) However, if the item or service is not covered by virtue of a national noncoverage policy in the Coverage Issues Manual and is the focus of a qualifying clinical trial, the routine costs of the clinical trial (as defined above) will be covered by Medicare but the noncovered item or service, itself, will not.

Requirements for Medicare Coverage of Routine Costs

Any clinical trial receiving Medicare coverage of routine costs must meet the following three requirements:

1. The subject or purpose of the trial must be the evaluation of an item or service that falls within a Medicare benefit category (e.g., physicians' service, durable medical equipment, diagnostic test) and is not statutorily excluded from coverage (e.g., cosmetic surgery, hearing aids).

2. The trial must not be designed exclusively to test toxicity or disease pathophysiology. It must have therapeutic intent.

3. Trials of therapeutic interventions must enroll patients with diagnosed disease rather than healthy volunteers. Trials of diagnostic interventions may enroll healthy patients in order to have a proper control group.

The three requirements above are insufficient by themselves to qualify a clinical trial for Medicare coverage of routine costs. Clinical trials also should have the following desirable characteristics; however, some trials, as described below, are presumed to meet these characteristics and are automatically qualified to receive Medicare coverage:

1. The principal purpose of the trial is to test whether the intervention potentially improves the participants' health outcomes;

2. The trial is well-supported by available scientific and medical information or it is intended to clarify or establish the health outcomes of interventions already in common clinical use;

3. The trial does not unjustifiably duplicate existing studies;

4. The trial design is appropriate to answer the research question being asked in the trial;

5. The trial is sponsored by a credible organization or individual capable of executing the proposed trial successfully;

6. The trial is in compliance with Federal regulations relating to the protection of human subjects; and

7. All aspects of the trial are conducted according to the appropriate standards of scientific integrity.

Qualification Process for Clinical Trials

Using the authority found in §1142 of the Act (cross-referenced in §1862(a)(1)(E) of the Act), the Agency for Healthcare Research and Quality (AHRQ) will convene a multi-agency Federal panel (the "panel") composed of representatives of the Department of Health and Human Services research agencies (National Institutes of Health (NIH), Centers for Disease Control and Prevention (CDC), the Food and Drug Administration (FDA), AHRQ, and the Office of Human Research Protection), and the research arms of the Department of Defense (DOD) and the Department of Veterans Affairs (VA) to develop qualifying criteria that will indicate a strong probability that a trial exhibits the desirable characteristics listed above. These criteria will be easily verifiable, and where possible, dichoto-mous. Trials that meet these qualifying criteria will receive Medicare cover-age of their associated routine costs. This panel is not reviewing or approv-ing individual trials. The multi-agency panel will meet periodically to review and evaluate the program and recommend any necessary refinements to CMS.

Clinical trials that meet the qualifying criteria will receive Medicare cover-age of routine costs after the trial's lead principal investigator certifies that the trial meets the criteria. This process will require the principal investiga-tor to enroll the trial in a Medicare clinical trials registry, currently under development.

Some clinical trials are automatically qualified to receive Medicare coverage of their routine costs because they have been deemed by AHRQ, in consul-tation with the other agencies represented on the multi-agency panel to be highly likely to have the above-listed seven desirable characteristics of clini-cal trials. The principal investigators of these automatically qualified trials do not need to certify that the trials meet the qualifying criteria, but must enroll the trials in the Medicare clinical trials registry for administrative purposes, once the registry is established.

Effective September 19, 2000, clinical trials that are deemed to be automatically qualified are:

1.   Trials funded by NIH, CDC, AHRQ, CMS, DOD, and VA;

2. Trials supported by centers or cooperative groups that are funded by the NIH, CDC, AHRQ, CMS, DOD and VA;

3. Trials conducted under an investigational new drug application (IND) reviewed by the FDA; and

4. Drug trials that are exempt from having an IND under 21 CFR 312.2(b)(1) will be deemed automatically qualified until the qualifying criteria are developed and the certification process is in place. At that time the principal investigators of these trials must certify that the trials meet the qualifying criteria in order to maintain Medicare coverage of routine costs. This certification process will only affect the future status of the trial and will not be used to retroactively change the earlier deemed status.

Medicare will cover the routine costs of qualifying trials that either have been deemed to be automatically qualified or have certified that they meet the qualifying criteria unless CMS's Chief Clinical Officer subsequently finds that a clinical trial does not meet the qualifying criteria or jeopardizes the safety or welfare of Medicare beneficiaries.

Should CMS find that a trial's principal investigator misrepresented that the trial met the necessary qualifying criteria in order to gain Medicare coverage of routine costs, Medicare coverage of the routine costs would be denied under §1862(a)(1)(E) of the Act. In the case of such a denial, the Medicare beneficiaries enrolled in the trial would not be held liable (i.e., would be held harmless from collection) for the costs consistent with the provisions of §1879, §1842(l), or §1834(j)(4) of the Act, as applicable. Where appropriate, the billing providers would be held liable for the costs and fraud investigations of the billing providers and the trial's principal investigator may be pursued.

Medicare regulations require Medicare+Choice (M+C) organizations to follow CMS's national coverage decisions. This NCD raises special issues that require some modification of most M+C organizations' rules governing provision of items and services in and out of network. The items and services covered under this NCD are inextricably linked to the clinical trials with which they are associated and cannot be covered outside of the context of those clinical trials. M+C organizations therefore must cover these services regardless of whether they are available through in-network providers. M+C organizations may have reporting requirements when enrollees participate in clinical trials, in order to track and coordinate their members' care, but cannot require prior authorization or approval. For the initial implementation, Medicare contractors will pay providers directly on a fee for service basis for covered clinical trial services for beneficiaries enrolled in M+C plans.

Source: CMS, www.cms.gov.